This report contains the collective views of an international group of experts and does not necessarily represent the decisions or the stated policy of the United Nations Environment Programme, the International Labour Organisation, or the World Health Organization

Environmental Health Criteria 60

PRINCIPLES AND METHODS FOR THE ASSESSMENT OF NEUROTOXICITY ASSOCIATED WITH EXPOSURE TO CHEMICALS

Published under the joint sponsorship of
the United Nations Environment Programme,
the International Labour Organisation,
and the World Health Organization

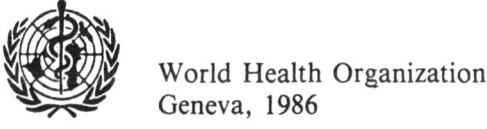

World Health Organization
Geneva, 1986

The International Programme on Chemical Safety (IPCS) is a joint venture of the United Nations Environment Programme, the International Labour Organisation, and the World Health Organization. The main objective of the IPCS is to carry out and disseminate evaluations of the effects of chemicals on human health and the quality of the environment. Supporting activities include the development of epidemiological, experimental laboratory, and risk-assessment methods that could produce internationally comparable results, and the development of manpower in the field of toxicology. Other activities carried out by IPCS include the development of know-how for coping with chemical accidents, coordination of laboratory testing and epidemiological studies, and promotion of research on the mechanisms of the biological action of chemicals.

ISBN 92 4 154260 8

©World Health Organization 1986

Reprinted 1992

Publications of the World Health Organization enjoy copyright protection in accordance with the provisions of Protocol 2 of the Universal Copyright Convention. For rights of reproduction or translation of WHO publications, in part or *in toto,* application should be made to the Office of Publications, World Health Organization, Geneva, Switzerland. The World Health Organization welcomes such applications.

The designations employed and the presentation of the material in this publication do not imply the expression of any opinion whatsoever on the part of the Secretariat of the World Health Organization concerning the legal status of any country, territory, city or area or of its authorities, or concerning the delimitation of its frontiers or boundaries.

The mention of specific companies or of certain manufacturers' products does not imply that they are endorsed or recommended by the World Health Organization in preference to others of a similar nature that are not mentioned. Errors and omissions excepted, the names of proprietary products are distinguished by initial capital letters.

ISSN 0250-863X
PRINTED IN FINLAND
DHSS — VAMMALA — 5500
92/9374 — VAMMALA — 500

CONTENTS

	Page
PRINCIPLES AND METHODS FOR THE ASSESSMENT OF NEUROTOXICITY ASSOCIATED WITH EXPOSURE TO CHEMICALS	

PREFACE 11

1. INTRODUCTION 13

    1.1 The importance of studying the nervous system . 13
        1.1.1 Methylmercury 14
        1.1.2 Carbon disulfide (CS_2) 16
    1.2 Need to establish a comprehensive strategy
        for neurotoxicity testing 18
    1.3 Scope of the book 19
    1.4 Purpose of the publication 20

2. GENERAL PRINCIPLES FOR THE ASSESSMENT OF TOXIC
    EFFECTS OF CHEMICALS ON THE NERVOUS SYSTEM 22

    2.1 Factors to be considered in the design of
        neurotoxicity studies 22
        2.1.1 General considerations 22
        2.1.2 Objectives 22
        2.1.3 Choice of animals 25
        2.1.4 Dosing regimen 27
        2.1.5 Functional reserve and adaptation 27
        2.1.6 Other factors 27
    2.2 Statistical analysis 28
        2.2.1 Type I and Type II errors 28
        2.2.2 Selection of the appropriate statistical
                test(s) 30

3. TEST METHODS IN BEHAVIOURAL TOXICOLOGY 32

    3.1 Introduction 32
    3.2 Classes of behaviour 33
        3.2.1 Respondent behaviour 33
        3.2.2 Operant behaviour 36
    3.3 Test methods 38
        3.3.1 General attributes of behavioural
              methods 38
              3.3.1.1 Sensitivity and specificity . . 38
              3.3.1.2 Validity 38
              3.3.1.3 Replicability 39
              3.3.1.4 Costs 39

		Page
	3.3.2 Primary tests	39
	3.3.2.1 Functional observation battery	39
	3.3.2.2 Motor activity	40
	3.3.3 Secondary tests	41
	3.3.3.1 Intermittent schedules of reinforcement	41
	3.3.3.2 Motor function	44
	3.3.3.3 Sensory function	45
	3.3.3.4 Cognitive function	47
	3.3.3.5 Eating and drinking behaviour	53
	3.3.3.6 Social behaviour	54
	3.3.4 Strengths and weaknesses of various methods	55
3.4	Research needs	56
	3.4.1 Compensatory mechanisms	56
	3.4.2 Method development and refinement	57

4. NEUROPHYSIOLOGICAL METHODS IN NEUROTOXICOLOGY 59

4.1	Introduction	59
4.2	Methods for evaluation of the peripheral nervous system	59
	4.2.1 Conduction velocity	59
	4.2.2 Peripheral nerve terminal function	60
	4.2.3 Electromyography (EMG)	61
	4.2.4 Spinal reflex excitability	61
4.3	Methods for evaluation of the autonomic nervous system	62
	4.3.1 Electrocardiography (EKG)	62
	4.3.2 Blood pressure	62
4.4	Methods for the evaluation of the central nervous system	63
	4.4.1 Spontaneous activity - electroencephalography (EEG)	63
	4.4.2 Sensory systems	64
	4.4.3 General excitability	65
	4.4.3.1 Convulsive phenomena	65
	4.4.3.2 Stimulation of the cerebral motor cortex	66
	4.4.3.3 Recovery functions	67
	4.4.4 Cognitive function	67
	4.4.5 Synaptic and membrane activity	67
4.5	Interpretation issues	67
4.6	Summary and conclusions	69

5. MORPHOLOGICAL METHODS 71

	Page
5.1 Introduction	71
5.1.1 Role of morphology	71
5.1.2 Basis for morphological assessment	71
5.2 The nervous system and toxic injuries	73
5.2.1 The nervous system	73
5.2.2 Cellular structure of the nervous system	74
5.2.3 Neurocellular reaction to injury	76
5.2.3.1 Biological principles	76
5.2.3.2 Neurons	77
5.2.3.3 Myelinating cells	78
5.3 Experimental design and execution	80
5.3.1 General principles and procedure	80
5.3.2 Gross morphology	81
5.3.3 The role of histology	81
5.3.3.1 Biological principles dictating tissue response	81
5.3.4 Use of controls	82
5.3.5 Pattern of response	83
5.3.6 Data acquired	83
5.4 Principles, limitations, and pitfalls of the morphological approach	85
5.4.1 Tissue state	85
5.4.2 Principles of fixation	85
5.4.3 Principles of tissue sampling	87
5.4.4 Preparation of tissue for examination	89
5.4.5 Recognition of artefact	91
5.4.6 Recognition of normal structural variations	91
5.4.7 Qualitative versus quantitative approaches	91
5.5 Specific procedures	92
5.5.1 Introduction	92
5.5.2 Primary methods	92
5.5.2.1 Formaldehyde/paraffin method	92
5.5.2.2 Glutaraldehyde/epoxy method	95
5.5.3 Special methods	96
5.5.3.1 Peripheral nerve microdissection	96
5.5.3.2 Frozen sections	97
5.5.3.3 Histochemical methods	98
5.5.3.4 Golgi method	99
5.5.3.5 Transmission electron microscopy	99
5.5.3.6 Other anatomical methods	99
5.6 Conclusions	100

			Page
6.	BIOCHEMICAL AND NEUROENDOCRINOLOGICAL METHODS		101
	6.1 Introduction		101
	6.2 Fractionation methods		102
		6.2.1 Brain dissection	102
		6.2.2 Isolation of specific cell types	103
		6.2.3 Subcellular fractionation	104
	6.3 DNA, RNA, and protein synthesis		106
	6.4 Lipids, glycolipids, and glycoproteins		108
	6.5 Neurotransmitters		110
		6.5.1 Synthesis/degradation	110
		6.5.2 Transport/release	111
		6.5.3 Binding	112
		6.5.4 Ion channels	113
		6.5.5 Cyclic nucleotides	115
		6.5.6 Summary of nerve terminal function	115
	6.6 Energy metabolism		115
	6.7 Biochemical correlates of axonal degeneration		116
	6.8 Neuroendocrine assessments		117
		6.8.1 Anterior pituitary hormones	117
		6.8.2 Disruption of neuroendocrine function	118
		6.8.2.1 Direct pituitary effects	118
		6.8.2.2 Peripheral target effects	119
		6.8.2.3 Disruption of hypothalamic control of pituitary secretions	120
		6.8.2.4 Other sites of action	121
		6.8.3 Sex differences	123
	6.9 Recommendations for future research		123
7.	CONCLUSIONS AND RECOMMENDATIONS		126
	REFERENCES		128

WHO TASK GROUP ON PRINCIPLES AND METHODS FOR THE ASSESSMENT OF NEUROTOXICITY ASSOCIATED WITH EXPOSURE TO CHEMICALS

Members

b   Dr M.B. Abou-Donia, Department of Pharmacology, Duke University Medical Center, Durham, North Carolina, USA

b,c   Dr W.K. Anger, Neurobehavioral Research Section, Division of Biomedical and Behavioral Science, National Institute for Occupational Safety and Health, Cincinatti, Ohio, USA

b,c   Dr G. Bignami, Section of Neurobehavioural Pathophysiology, Laboratory of Organ and System Pathophysiology, High Institute of Health, Rome, Italy

b   Dr T.J. Bonashevskaya, Sysin Institute of General and Community Hygiene, Moscow, USSR

b   Dr E. Bonilla, Institute of Clinical Research, Faculty of Medicine, University of Zulia, Maracaibo, Venezuela

b,c   Professor J. Cavanagh, West Norwood, London, England (Rapporteur[b,c])

b   Dr V.A. Colotla, National Autonomous University, City University, Coyoacan, Mexico

b   Dr I. Desi, Division of Toxicology, National Institute of Hygiene, Budapest, Hungary

a   Dr L. Di Giamberardino, Département de Biologie, Commissariat à l'Energie Atomique, Centre d'Etudes Nucléaires de Saclay, Gif-sur-Yvette, France

b   Dr S. Frankova, Institute of Psychology, Czechoslovak Academy of Sciences, Prague, Czechoslovakia

b   Dr E. Frantik, Institute of Hygiene and Epidemiology, Prague, Czechoslovakia

c   Dr. I. Goto, Department of Neurology, Neurological Institute, Faculty of Medicine, Kyushu University, Higashiku, Fukuoka, Japan

b,c   Professor Dr M. Hasan, Brain Research Centre, J.N. Medical College, Aligharh Muslim University, Aligharh, India

b   Dr L. Hinkova, Institute of Hygiene and Occupational Health, Sofia, Bulgaria

a,b,c   Associate Professor Dr M. Horvath, Institute of Hygiene and Epidemiology, Prague, Czechoslovakia (Vice-Chairman[c])

c   Professor A. Korczyn, Neurology Department, Tel Aviv Medical Centre, Tel Aviv University, Tel Aviv, Israel

b   Dr N.N. Litvinov, Sysin Institute of General and Community Hygiene, Moscow, USSR

Members (contd).

a,b   Professor R.V. Merkureva, Departmen of Medical Biological Research, Sysin Institute of General and Community Hygiene, Moscow, USSR (Vice-Chairman<u>a</u>)

a,b,c   Dr C. Mitchell, Laboratory of Behavioural and Neurological Toxicology, National Institute of Environmental Health Sciences, Research Triangle Park, North Carolina, USA (Chairman<u>a</u>,<u>b</u>,<u>c</u>)

b,c   Professor J.E. Murad, Medical School and Chairman, Al. Ezequiel Dins, 275, Drugs Orientation Centre, Belo Horizonte, Brazil

b,c   Professor O.B. Osuntokun, Department of Medicine, University of Ibadan, WHO Collaborating Centre for Research and Training in Neurosciences, University of Ibadan, Nigeria

a,b,c   Dr L. Reiter, Division of Neurotoxicology (MD-74B), US Environmental Protection Agency, Health Effects Research Laboratory, Research Triangle Park, North Carolina, USA

b   Dr D.C. Rice, Toxicology Research Division, Food Directorate, Health Protection Branch, Department of National Health and Welfare, Tunney's Pasture, Ottawa, Ontario, Canada

b,c   Dr M. Rudnev, Kiev Research Institute of General and Communal Hygiene, Kiev, USSR

c   Dr M. Ruscak, Centre of Physiological Sciences, Slovak Academy of Sciences, Bratislava, Czechoslovakia

a   Dr H. Savolainen, Institute of Occupational Health, Helsinki, Finland (Rapporteur)

b,c   Professor V. Schreiber, Laboratory for Endodrinology, Faculty of Medicine, Charles University, Prague, Czechoslovakia

b,c   Professor P. Spencer, Institute of Neurotoxicology, Albert Einstein College of Medicine, New York, USA

b   Dr T. Tanimura, Department of Anatomy, Kinki University School of Medicine, Osaka, Japan (invited, but could not attend)

b,c   Dr H. Tilson, Laboratory of Behavioural and Neurological Toxicology, National Institute of Environmental Health Sciences, Research Triangle Park, North Carolina, USA

b,c   Dr L. Uphouse, Department of Biology, Texas Woman's University, Denton, Texas, USA

b,c   Dr T. Vergieva, Department of Toxicology, Institute of Hygiene and Occupational Health, Sofia, Bulgaria

c   Professor D. Warburton, Psychopharmacology Group, Early, Reading, United Kingdom

Members (contd).

a,b   Dr G. Winneke, Institute of Environmental Hygiene, University of Düsseldorf, Düsseldorf, Federal Republic of Germany

b   Dr V.G. Zilov, I.M. Sechnov Medical Institute, Department of Normal Physiology, Moscow, USSR (Vice-Chairman[b])

Secretariat

c   Dr G. Becking, International Programme on Chemical Safety, World Health Organization, Research Triangle Park, North Carolina, USA

a   Dr C.L. Bolis, Neurosciences Programme, World Health Organization, Geneva, Switzerland

a   Dr A. David, Office of Occupational Health, World Health Organization, Geneva, Switzerland

a,b,c   Dr M. Draper, International Programme on Chemical Safety, World Health Organization, Geneva, Switzerland

b   Dr M. Gounar, International Programme on Chemical Safety, World Health Organization, Geneva, Switzerland

a   Mr E. Hellen, Occupational Safety and Health Branch, International Labour Organisation, Geneva, Switzerland

a   Dr A.I. Koutcherenko, International Register for Potentially Toxic Chemicals, United Nations Environment Programme, Geneva, Switzerland

a   Dr M. Mercier, International Programme on Chemical Safety, World Health Organization, Geneva, Switzerland

b   Dr L.A. Moustafa, International Programme on Chemical Safety, World Health Organization, Research Triangle Park, North Carolina, USA

a   Dr J. Parizek, International Programme on Chemical Safety, World Health Organization, Geneva, Switzerland (Secretary)

a   Dr J. Purswell, Section on Hygiene, International Labour Organisation, Geneva, Switzerland

a   Dr C. Satkunananthan, International Programme on Chemical Safety, World Health Organization, Geneva, Switzerland (Temporary Adviser)

a   Dr C. Xintaras, Office of Occupational Health, World Health Organization, Geneva, Switzerland

---

a   Preparatory consultation, Geneva, 14-16 September 1981.
b   First Task Group meeting, Moscow, 1-7 June 1983.
c   Second Task Group meeting, Prague, 17-21 September 1984.

NOTE TO READERS OF THE CRITERIA DOCUMENTS

Every effort has been made to present information in the criteria documents as accurately as possible without unduly delaying their publication. In the interest of all users of the environmental health criteria documents, readers are kindly requested to communicate any errors that may have occurred to the Manager of the International Programme on Chemical Safety, World Health Organization, Geneva, Switzerland, in order that they may be included in corrigenda, which will appear in subsequent volumes.

* * *

PREFACE

The need for generally accepted scientific principles and requirements in all areas of toxicology particularly applies to the newly developed field of neurotoxicology. Methods continue to be developed in isolation, and the comparability of results is often in doubt. Furthermore, until scientific principles have been agreed on, internationally accepted strategies to test the effects of chemicals on the many functions of the mammalian nervous system will not be developed. At the suggestion of the two participating institutions (Sysin Institute of General and Community Hygiene, USSR, and the National Institute of Environmental Health Sciences, USA), the International Programme on Chemical Safety (IPCS) undertook a study of the principles and methods used to study the effects of chemicals on the nervous system (neurotoxicology) in order to lay the foundations for further developments in this important area of toxicology. The publication of the results of the study in a monograph seemed the most effective means of achieving this goal.

Members of an International Task Group of experts from 18 countries generously devoted much time to the preparation of the monograph, and the IPCS wishes to express its deep gratitude to all the members of the Task Group for their efforts.

The scope and plans for the development of the monograph were discussed at a consultation, chaired by Dr C.L. Mitchell with Dr R.V. Merkureva as Vice-Chairman. Representatives from the IPCS institutions that had expressed a particular interest in the assessment of neurotoxic effects of chemicals attended the meeting at the invitation of the Manager, IPCS, Dr M. Mercier. The following institutions were represented: National Institute of Environmental Health Sciences (NIEHS), Research Triangle Park, North Carolina, USA; Sysin Institute, Academy of Medical Sciences, Moscow, USSR; Institute of Hygiene and Epidemiology, Czechoslovak Academy of Sciences, Prague, Czechoslovakia; US Environmetal Protection Agency (US EPA), Health Effects Research Laboratories, Research Triangle Park, North Carolina, USA; Atomic Energy Commission, Department of Biology, Gif-sur-Yvette, France; Institute of Occupational Health, Helsinki, Finland; and Institute of Environmental Hygiene, University of Düsseldorf, Federal Republic of Germany. It was agreed that nine background papers would be used as the basis for the preparation of sections in a monograph reviewing the principles and methods for the evaluation of effects on the nervous system associated with exposure to chemicals.

On 1-7 June 1983, the first meeting of the Task Group was convened in Moscow, hosted by the USSR Ministry of Health, the

USSR Commission for UNEP, and the Centre for International Projects, GKNT. The Sysin Institute of General and Community Hygiene collaborated in the preparations for this meeting. Dr S.N. Bajbakov, Director, Centre of International Projects, GKNT, formally opened the meeting and Dr A.M. Pisarev, USSR Ministry of Health and Dr N.N. Litvinov of the Sysin Institute added greetings to the Task Group. It was agreed that Dr C.L. Mitchell would be Chairman and Dr V.G. Zilov, Vice-Chairman. Dr J.B. Cavanagh was asked to be Rapporteur of the meeting.

The scope and content of ten background papers made available by the Secretariat were discussed thoroughly by the experts, and agreement was reached on the appropriate sections needed. After a detailed discussion on the issues to be addressed in each section, the meeting divided into five working groups to draft the texts for the following sections: General Principles, Morphology/Pathology, Biochemistry, Neuroendocrinology, Neurophysiology, and Behaviour. At the end of the meeting, most of the text was completed, and Dr Mitchell was asked to act as an overall editor to assist the Working Group leaders in completing their sections.

A revised text was submitted to the Task Group before its second meeting, held in Prague on 17-21 September 1984. Dr C.L. Mitchell was again asked to be Chairman and Dr M. Horvath, Vice-Chairman. Dr J. Cavanagh was appointed Rapporteur. The meeting was hosted by the Ministry of Health of the Czech Socialist Republic, Prague, and Professor Dr D. Zuskova welcomed the experts on behalf of the Minister of Health. The final text for the document was agreed upon by the end of the meeting. Dr Mitchell was asked to continue as overall editor to ensure the incorporation of all material discussed at the meeting, including the appropriate references.

The International Programme on Chemical Safety wishes to acknowledge the valuable help provided by many scientists who were not members of the Task Group, and, in particular, that of Dr R. Dyer (Neurophysiology), Dr R. McPhail and the late Dr P. Ruppert (Behaviour) of the US EPA, and Dr T. Damstra (Neurochemistry) of the National Institute of Environmental Health Sciences.

* * *

Partial financial support for the publication of this criteria document was kindly provided by the United States Department of Health and Human Services, through a contract from the National Institute of Environmental Health Sciences, Research Triangle Park, North Carolina, USA - a WHO Collaborating Centre for Environmental Health Effects. The United Kingdom Department of Health and Social Security generously covered the costs of printing.

1. INTRODUCTION

Interest in nervous system toxicology has been growing in recent years, not only because of increased public concern over the impact of toxic agents on human health and the quality of life, but also because the nervous system has been shown to be particularly vulnerable to chemical insult. Thus, there has been an increased demand for improved methods for the detection of neurotoxic effects and the assessment of health risks within the field of occupational and environmental health and safety research related to the science known as "Neurotoxicology" (Spencer & Schaumburg, 1980; O'Donoghue, 1985).

Neurotoxicology includes studies on the actions of chemical, biological, and certain physical agents that produce adverse effects on the nervous system and/or behaviour during development and at maturity. Toxic disorders of the nervous system of human beings and animals may occur following abuse of such substances as ethanol, inhalants, narcotics, therapeutic drugs, products or components of living organisms (e.g., bacteria, fungi, plants, animals), chemicals designed to affect certain organisms (e.g., pest-control products), industrial chemicals, chemical warfare agents, additives and natural components of food, raw materials for perfumes, and certain other types of chemicals encountered in the environment.

This document is intended to aid in the design and assessment of studies concerned with exploring the association between exposure to chemicals and the development of adverse neurobehavioural changes. The emphasis is on animals as systems to model and predict adverse reactions of the human nervous system to exogenous chemicals.

1.1 The Importance of Studying the Nervous System

The brain is an extremely complex organ, the function of which is to receive and integrate signals and then to respond appropriately, to maintain bodily functions. It supports a diversity of complex processes including cognition, awareness, memory, and language. Sexual behaviour, locomotion, and the use of a vast array of tools ranging from the slingshot to the microcomputer, suggest the range of responses available to the human organism. Moreover, the nervous system is influenced by the functioning of other organ systems (e.g., hepatic, cardiovascular, and endocrine systems). Thus, toxicant-induced alterations in any of these organ systems can be reflected in changes in neurobehavioural output. This fact alone suggests that nervous system function should be among the first to be thoroughly assessed in cases of exposure to known or potentially hazardous agents.

Major outbreaks of neurotoxicity in human populations of various sizes have emphasized the importance of neurotoxicology as an independent discipline. Poisoning episodes have resulted from exposures in the environment (e.g., methylmercury, lead), at the work-place (e.g., hexanes, carbon disulfide, leptophos, chlordecone), as well as from food toxins (cassava) and food contaminants (triorthocresyl phosphate (TOCP)). There are numerous sources of reference dealing with chemicals reported to produce behavioural and neurological effects in human beings and laboratory animals including Horvath (1973), Xintaras et al. (1974), Weiss & Laties (1975), Spencer & Schaumburg (1980), and O'Donoghue (1985). These references should be consulted by the reader unfamiliar with this area of toxicology.

At present, it is not possible to give a precise estimate of the number of chemicals that exert behavioural or neurotoxic effects. Anger & Johnson (1985) list more than 850 chemicals that have been reported to produce such effects. Anger (1984) states that, of the 588 chemicals listed in the 1982 edition of the American Conference of Governmental Industrial Hygienists publication "Threshold Limit Values for Chemical Substances and Physical Agents in the Workroom Environment", 167 (29%) "have threshold limit values (recommended exposure maxima) based, at least in part, on direct neurological or behavioural effects, or on factors associated with the nervous system (viz., cholinesterase inhibition)." The neurotoxic properties of chemicals have been identified because of the conspicuous nature of severe signs and symptoms. It is not known how often insidious problems of neurotoxicity may lie undetected because the effects are incorrectly attributed to other conditions (e.g., advancing age, mood disorders) or misdiagnosed. The early and incipient stages of intoxications produced by environmental agents are frequently marked by vagueness and ambiguity (Mello, 1975; US NAS, 1975), and many complaints are subjective (e.g., fatigue, anxiety, irritability, lethargy, headache, weakness, depression). Thus, the potential is large for the occurrence of subtle, undetected effects, which nonetheless have an important bearing on the quality of life.

The following examples illustrate the types of neurotoxic outbreaks that have occurred and exemplify the usefulness of animal models to further characterize this neurotoxicity.

1.1.1 Methylmercury

The neurotoxicity of mercury compounds has received world-wide attention for centuries (Hunter et al., 1940).

However, it was not until the outbreak of methylmercury poisoning in Minamata, Japan in the 1950s that the extreme toxicological consequences of human exposure were fully recognized (Takeuchi, 1968). During this outbreak of poisoning, thousands of inhabitants were exposed to methylmercury. The source of exposure was found to be industrial effluent that contained large amounts of mercury. The mercury made its way into Minamata Bay where it was converted to methylmercury by marine biota. This accumulated in fish and shellfish, which were eventually consumed by the local residents. This consumption of contaminated seafood continued for several years and resulted in hundreds of reported cases of methylmercury poisoning. Since that time, methylmercury poisoning has been referred to as "Minamata Disease".

A second major outbreak of methylmercury poisoning occurred in Iraq during 1971-72 (Bakir et al., 1973). In this case, the source of exposure was the ingestion of seed grain treated with a methylmercury fungicide; the grain had been ground into flour to make bread. Approximately 6500 people were hospitalized due to poisoning, and at least 400 died.

The clinical manifestations of methylmercury poisoning are quite extensive and include disturbances in sensory, motor, and cognitive functions. The earliest complaints are associated with sensory loss in the extremities, perioral numbness and concentric constriction of the visual fields, followed by the development of ataxic gait, dyarthria, incoordination, intention tremor, hearing problems, and muscle weakness (Takeuchi et al., 1979). Mental disturbances, as well as alterations in taste, smell, and salivation have also been reported (Takeuchi, 1968; Chang, 1977, 1980; Reuhl & Chang, 1979, Takeuchi et al., 1979).

The pattern of sensory neural damage in the monkey resembles that of man. Visual system deficits in primates include constriction of visual fields, deficit in scotopic (low light) vision (Evans et al., 1975), and deficit in ability to detect flicker (Merigan, 1980). Spatial visual function was impaired in monkeys dosed from birth (Rice & Gilbert, 1982). Hypoesthesia (impaired sense of touch) has been reported in the monkey (Evans et al., 1975) as well as man (Hunter et al., 1940). Moreover, the body burden at which signs are observed in primates is similar to that reported for human beings.

In rodents, neurobehavioural research on methylmercury has concentrated primarily on an evaluation of the later motor effects, but some of the sensory deficits have not been found (Shaw et al., 1975, 1980; Evans et al., 1977). Several investigators have observed a progressive weakness of the hindlimbs followed by decrease in forelimb function (Diamond &

Sleight, 1972; Klein et al., 1972; Herman et al., 1973; Snyder & Braun, 1977; Ohi et al., 1978). Grip strength was reported to be reduced in rats following long-term dosing with methylmercury (Pryor et al., 1983). Decreased motor activity in mice exposed to methylmercury in the drinking-water was reported by MacDonald & Harbison (1977), but horizontally-directed motor activity did not appear to be markedly affected by repeated exposure to methylmercury (Salvaterra et al., 1973; Morganti et al., 1976). Responsiveness to noxious stimuli was reportedly intact in methylmercury-exposed rats, even in the presence of gross neuromotor deficits (Herman et al., 1973; Salvaterra et al., 1973). Similarly, Pryor et al. (1983) did not observe any significant alteration in startle responsiveness to an acoustic stimulus in methylmercury-exposed rats. Finally, in an attempt to investigate the effects of mercury on development, prepubescent rats were exposed to a single dose of methylmercury. Ability to learn an active avoidance response at 70 days of age was impaired (Reuhl & Chang, 1979).

1.1.2 Carbon disulfide (CS_2)

Carbon disulfide (CS_2) is a volatile solvent that has been used for a variety of industrial purposes. Since its discovery in 1776, there have been numerous examples of CS_2-induced neurotoxicity. Many cases of human CS_2 poisoning occurred in the viscose industry during and after the second world war and consisted of various neurological and behavioural effects. According to Braceland (1942), the psychological effects consisted of personality changes, irritability, memory deficits, insomnia, bad dreams, decreased libido, and constant fatigue.

Paraesthesia and dysesthesia from CS_2 exposure tend to occur in a "stocking and glove" distribution characteristic of peripheral nerve injury and indeed Seppalainen et al. (1972) reported a slowing of motor conduction in peripheral nerves. Various sensory alterations have been reported following CS_2 exposure, particularly in vision. Central field loss, disturbances in colour vision, enlargement of the blind spot, and reduction in peripheral vision have been reported. Alterations in auditory, vestibular, and olfactory senses have also been reported (Wood, 1981).

While there have been few studies that have attempted to quantify the sensory and psychological effects of CS_2 in laboratory animals (Wood, 1981), the neuropathological changes and effects on motor behaviour have been extensively studied. CS_2 produces filamentous inclusions in axons in both the central and peripheral nervous systems. Experimental CS_2 neuropathy consisting of weakness or loss of power in the limbs, depressed reflexes, and general behavioural suppression has been reported in dogs (Lewey, 1941), rabbits (Seppalainen & Linnoila, 1975), and rats (Frantik, 1970; Lukas, 1970). Tilson et al. (1979b) reported decreases in grip strength and motor activity in rats following CS_2 exposure; Horvath (1973) found decreases in motor activity in rats following exposure to high concentrations of CS_2, but motor activity increased following exposure to low concentrations.

The cases illustrated above are unfortunately typical in that the neurotoxicity of the chemicals was first discovered when human beings exposed to them became ill. Later, research using animal models in a controlled setting provided experimental evidence that the chemical believed to have caused the illness in the human population produced similar effects in animals. One purpose of this book is to provide the background through which this process can be reversed; i.e., the chemical can be tested in an animal model before human beings become overexposed, seriously ill, or irreversibly harmed by it.

There are a few examples where this principle has been put into practice. Some compounds have been discovered to be neurotoxic in animals and, as a result, further human exposure has been discontinued. Other chemicals, shown to be neurotoxic for animals, have only later been discovered to produce comparable disorders in human beings.

The former is illustrated by Musk Tetralin, a synthetic musk introduced in 1955 as a raw material and as an artificial flavouring substance. Apparently, the minimal acute toxicity testing in use at that time suggested that the compound was acceptable for human consumption. After 20 years of widespread use in the domestic environment, a new set of long-term animal toxicity studies showed that the substance was a potent neurotoxin inducing behavioural changes and irreversible structural damage throughout the nervous system of dermally- or orally-exposed animals (Spencer et al., 1980).

Two examples illustrate that experimental animal studies may reveal the neurotoxic properties of substances before they are discovered in human beings. One concerns aluminium, a substance that was shown to induce central nervous system toxicity in animals as early as 1886. Subsequent studies confirmed this, before the first case of suspected human aluminum encephalopathy was reported in 1962. With the introduction of aluminium-containing phosphate-binding gels for the haemodialysis of individuals with kidney dysfunction, large numbers of treated patients developed a progressive dementing illness that often proved fatal (Crapper & DeBoni, 1980). Another recent example of this phenomenon concerns the peripheral neurotoxicity of megavitamin doses of pyridoxine phosphate (vitamin B_6), recently reported in human beings taking the drug in prescribed amounts for therapeutic purposes (Schaumburg, 1982). The clinical neurological syndrome had been reproduced in animals some 40 years previously and would not have been recognized in human beings but for more recent experimental animal work that had highlighted the surprising neurotoxic potential of this essential nutrient (Krinke et al., 1981).

Both examples demonstrate the power of animal studies in predicting human neurotoxicity and both illustrate the need for the medical world to pay close attention to discoveries in experimental neurotoxicology. With the further refinement and validation of methods used in this discipline, it should be possible to discover many other potentially harmful agents, presently in use, and to prevent new compounds with neurotoxic properties from reaching the human environment. Compounds that have been identified, through various types of research, are listed in Table 1 according to important nervous system targets.

1.2 Need to Establish A Comprehensive Strategy for Neurotoxicity Testing

The need to establish a comprehensive strategy for neurotoxicity testing is made clear by estimates recently provided by the US EPA Office of Toxic Substances. In the USA alone, between 40 000 and 60 000 chemicals are currently in commercial use; furthermore, approximately 1000 new chemicals are introduced into commerce each year (Reiter, 1980). It is not surprising that few or no toxicological data exist for many of these chemicals. Therefore, any toxicity testing strategy intended for general use must be flexible enough to evaluate a wide variety of chemicals and chemical classes and must be able to take into account the potential for chemical interaction, as most people are exposed to combinations of chemicals. The toxicological data that are available for a given chemical will influence testing requirements for that chemical. For example, the desired approach will depend on whether the investigation has been initiated to evaluate the toxicity of the chemical prior to its commercial use or to confirm reports of chemically-induced disease in man.

Risk from exposure to a toxic substance is a function of both the intrinsic toxicity of the chemical and the human exposure pattern. These factors will influence where it enters the testing scheme; its potency and the human exposure pattern will influence the extent to which testing must be pursued. In both cases, steps must be incorporated that facilitate decision-making about acceptance, rejection, or continuation of testing. However, the eventual goal is to

Table 1. Illustrative manifestations of human neurotoxicity

Function affected	Manifestation	Chemical example
Sensorium change	irritability	carbon disulfide
	apathy/lethargy	carbon monoxide
	attention difficulty	anticholinesterases
	illusions, delusions, hallucinations	ergot
	dementia	aluminium
	depression, euphoria	ozocerite
	stupor, coma	dicyclopentadiene
Sensory special	Abnormalities of:	
	smell	cadmium
	vision	methanol
	taste	selenium
	hearing	toluene
	balance	methyl nitrite
Somatosensory	skin senses (e.g., numbness, pain)	trichloroethylene thallium
	proprioception	acrylamide
Motor	muscle weakness: paralysis, spasticity, rigidity	organophosphates Lathyrus sativus methyl phenyl tetrahydropyridine
	tremor	chlordecone
	dystonia	manganese
	incoordination	organomercury
	hyperactivity	lead
	myoclonus	toluene
	fasciculation	anticholinesterases
	cramps	styrene
	seizures, convulsions	acetonitrile
Autonomic	Abnormalities of:	
	sweating	acrylamide
	temperature control	chlordane
	gastrointestinal function	lead
	appetite, body-weight, cardiovascular control, urination	dinitrobenzene vocor dimethylamino-propionitrile
	sexual function	β-chloroprene

understand the mechanism(s) by which chemicals adversely alter nervous system function.

1.3 Scope of the Book

Emphasis in this book is placed on animal test data. An important role of the toxicologist, of course, is to provide data that can be used for quantitative estimation of the risks associated with exposure of human populations to toxic chemicals. Even in extensively explored areas such as carcinogenesis, risk assessment is an extremely difficult undertaking for which there is no concise research strategy. A major problem in dealing with most chemicals is that the available toxicological data base concerning precise information on human health effects is relatively sparse. The neurotoxicological data base is no exception in this respect; in particular, adequate human behavioural data are available for only a few chemicals (Anger & Johnson, 1985). Furthermore, a number of experimental problems inherent in most published human studies cloud interpretation of data from these studies. Perhaps the most serious problem is that of adequately defining the exposure level (dose) in human populations, a critical factor in risk assessment. Other factors that influence behavioural measures include sex, age, cultural variables, disease states, and possible exposure to additional toxic substances (Johnson & Anger, 1983). As these critical variables cannot be adequately controlled in human field studies, in all or even most cases, the neurotoxicologist must rely to a great extent on animal test data to establish accurate dose-effect relationships.

A word should be said about related and important areas excluded from this publication. Developmental and human neurotoxicology are not discussed in detail, since they have already been addressed in other publications of the World Health Organization (WHO, 1984; WHO, in preparation). The usefulness of tissue culture techniques will be considered in a future publication. The closely related area of psychopharmacology, which assesses the effects of drugs on the nervous system, is not within the scope of this document and has been addressed in other publications (CIOMS, 1983). However, many of the methods identified in this manuscript have been used in this area.

The very important role played by the autonomic nervous system in the regulation of many physiological processes is well recognized (Dyck et al., 1984). However, it has not been possible to discuss in any detail the principles of the methods available to study the effects of chemicals on this system. A detailed discussion of such methods will be presented in a WHO publication that is in preparation and deals with methods for the assessment of toxicity from exposure to chemicals.

1.4 Purpose of the Publication

Given the magnitude of the problem and the potential for subtle damage to the nervous system, there is a pressing need to assess the behavioural and neurological effects of the mass of chemicals found in the work-place and the ambient environment.

The purpose of this book is to provide an overview of the principles of neurobehavioural assessment and to identify methods that have been successfully applied to the study of neurotoxicity in the past. These methods, which may eventually be modified or supplemented by other better methods, have been generally established and can be relied on to provide an assessment of chemicals for their neurotoxicity. The references for each method can be consulted for further details.

The book is divided into five sections. The first deals with principles of assessment, and the remaining sections deal with methods in the four major research disciplines that contribute substantially to the assessment of the neurotoxicity of chemicals found in the occupational or community environment. Each discipline is not in a comparable stage of development as it relates to neurotoxic assessment of environmental chemicals. Behavioural and neurophysiological methods have been extensively applied, but there is limited agreement on which of the many methods described are the most appropriate for the initial screening of an unknown chemical and, thus, the approach of tiered testing is suggested or general guidelines are given for selecting methods. On the other hand, the neuromorphological section presents a relatively more methodological approach to the neuropathological assessment of nervous tissue that has been validated in other areas of research, recognizing that it is the experience of the neuropathologist that is critical to an adequate assessment rather than the test methods, as in the sections mentioned above. Finally, the section on endocrinological and biochemical methods reflects the fact that these methods have been applied far less to the neurotoxic assessment of environmental contaminants. However, their inclusion is important because of the critical role they play in exposure monitoring and the elucidation of mechanisms.

2. GENERAL PRINCIPLES FOR THE ASSESSMENT OF TOXIC EFFECTS OF CHEMICALS ON THE NERVOUS SYSTEM

2.1 Factors to be Considered in the Design of Neurotoxicity Studies

2.1.1 General considerations

Many factors must be taken into consideration with regard to any toxicology study. These include the choice and number of animals, dosage, route and duration of administration, metabolism and pharmacokinetics, and testing procedures. These have been discussed in detail elsewhere (US NAS/NRC, 1970; US NAS, 1975; WHO, 1978) and the various reference sources should be consulted, as only aspects of special relevance to neurotoxicology will be emphasized here.

The nervous system is protected from undesirable external influences by both physical and chemical barriers. This protection, however, is not complete. The blood-brain barrier has an important function in preserving the chemical constitution of the nervous system, but some noxious substances, particularly those that are lipid soluble, may still cross it. Another mode of entry is by uptake into the peripheral terminals of nerves, which may then transfer the substances into their cell bodies in the central nervous system through retrograde axonal flow. Such a mechanism operates for substances as remote as tetanus toxin and some viruses. The peripheral nervous system is, of course, more likely to be exposed to neurotoxicity. The neurons of the autonomic nervous system and the sensory ganglia are outside the blood-brain barrier, as are small regions of the CNS, circumventricular organs (e.g., area postrema) and, to a limited extent, the retina.

As might be expected, the nervous system may be particularly vulnerable either during development or in senescence. Some aspects of this have been alluded to elsewhere (WHO, 1984). Physical changes or the presence of toxins may also disrupt the blood-brain barrier and, thus, allow substances normally excluded from the brain to reach and affect it adversely.

2.1.2 Objectives

The objectives of neurotoxicity testing are to:

(a) identify whether the nervous system is altered by the toxicant (detection);

(b) characterize the nervous system alterations associated with exposure;

(c) ascertain whether the nervous system is the primary target for the chemical; and

(d) determine dose- and time-effect relationships aimed at establishing a no-observed-adverse-effect level.

In a sense, these objectives translate into a series of questions about the toxicity of a chemical, and achieving them requires behavioural, neurophysiological, biochemical, and neuropathological information.

When faced with a chemical for which no toxicological data are available, the first question is whether the nervous system is or is not affected by the chemical. This represents the most fundamental level of investigation and entails procedures that "screen" for neurotoxicity. Such tests must not only forecast the potential of a substance to produce adverse effects, but must also be simple, rapid, and economical to administer. Once a chemical is known to produce neurotoxic effects, further studies must be performed in order to characterize the nature and mechanism of the alterations. These studies explore the consequences of toxicant exposure and give an indication of whether or not the nervous system is the primary target organ.

Many functions are mediated by unique neural substrates, and chemicals may produce selective effects. Thus, it is important to use a variety of tests that measure different functions, in order to maximize the probability of detecting a toxic effect. It is clear that the methods used may differ depending on the following factors:

(a) the objective of the study;

(b) the age of the animal; and

(c) the species examined.

If the objective of the study is to provide an initial evaluation of the effect of a new substance on the nervous system, the methods used may differ considerably from those used when a great deal is known about a substance, and its mechanism of action is being investigated, or environmental or occupational standards are being set for acceptable levels in the biosphere. If the objective is to contribute substantively to the overall toxic risk assessment for the chemical, the methods used should attempt to model human disease states. Thus, it is important that the purpose of the study is clear to both the investigator and the evaluator. In many situations, the evaluation of reference substances in the same protocols will help determine the specificity and validity of the observed changes. It also makes it possible to evaluate the relative potency of different chemicals (Horvath & Frantik, 1973), and this is always essential for the novice investigator or for the investigator using a new technique.

Although certain chemicals produce selective damage in the nervous system, a more common finding is one of widespread damage and disruption of a variety of functions. Ideally, characterization of such generalized neurotoxicity by a variety of methods will establish a profile of the disrupted functions.

Once a chemical has been identified as neurotoxic, the next objective is to determine dose-effect and time-effect relationships. One aim of these studies is to establish no-observed-adverse-effect levels, but to prove that a certain dose produces no effect may require a very large number of experimental animals (Dews, 1982). To be useful in risk assessment, threshold determinations must be obtained by the most sensitive tests available. For example, as the toxic effects of methylmercury became known, studies using subhuman primates began to focus on its effects on the visual system. Alterations in visual function in monkeys following methylmercury exposure has now been well documented using sophisticated visual psychophysical techniques (Evans et al., 1975).

The question of how to define toxicity is of critical importance for the ultimate goal of risk assessment and the establishment of hygienic standards. Considerable controversy exists concerning what constitutes an adverse effect in toxicology. According to one view, any evidence of a behavioural or biological change is considered to be an adverse effect. According to others, evidence is required of both an irreversible decrement in the ability of the organism to maintain homeostasis and/or an enhanced susceptibility to the deleterious effects of other environmental influences. In this latter view, differentiation between "nonadversive" and "adverse" effects requires considerable knowledge of the importance of reversible changes and subtle departures from "normal" behaviour, physiology, biochemistry, and morphology in terms of the organism's overall economy of life, ability to adapt to other stresses, and their possible effects on life span (WHO, 1978). Real or potential risks to the nervous system are difficult to assess because of its complexity. Some of the problems in assessment are associated with the wide variations that can occur but are still considered to be within the "normal" range. Some are associated with the plasticity of the nervous system. Other problems in assessment are related to incomplete understanding of what is being measured by certain tests. It is clear, therefore, that no single test will suffice to examine the functional capacity of the nervous system.

The above comments suggest tiered testing approaches, such as those recommended in the section on behavioural methods, where a variety of testing schemes, ranging from simple to complex, have been proposed (Pavlenko, 1975; US NAS, 1975; Tilson & Cabe, 1978). Such schemes typically begin with simple, rapid, inexpensive tests for detecting the presence of neurobehavioural effects. The tests in successive stages are designed to answer increasingly specific questions about the toxicity of the chemical. Each stage should also incorporate decision points as to whether the available information is sufficient for determining the toxicity of the chemical. When combined with estimates of potential exposure of human populations, this information can provide a basis for evaluating the justification for proceeding to the next level of testing. The advantage of the tiered approach is that decisions are made at each level of testing and, therefore, scarce resources are directed towards chemicals for which the greatest hazard or risk potential exists.

Obviously, the amount of available information about the substance will determine the level at which the chemical will enter this testing scheme. Another inherent assumption is that a chemical's pattern of use, in combination with its toxic potency, will be considered in any decision about further testing. Testing requirements for a chemical that is indigenous the environment and to which large segments of the population are exposed will require extensive investigation leading, ideally, to determination of the no-observed-adverse-effect level. This information is extremely useful to governmental agencies responsible for setting exposure or hygienic standards. On the other hand, compounds that are being introduced into commerce and/or for which the projected exposure is limited may require less testing.

2.1.3   Choice of animals

For obvious reasons of safety and ethics, it is necessary to use animals in toxicity assessments. However, the extrapolation of animal toxicological data to human beings is always tenuous and should be carried out with caution. In preliminary mass screening of known or suspected environmental toxicants, there are economic factors that must be taken into account. It is also important that there be adequate anatomical, physiological, pharmacological, and toxicological data bases on the species chosen for study, so that meaningful interpretations of effects can be made and appropriate hypotheses about mechanisms and loci of action can be framed. For these reasons, the mouse or rat is usually preferred in a preliminary screen, though the rodent differs from man in many significant ways. For more detailed studies, other species may provide a more appropriate model. For example, the adult chicken is the animal of choice to test organophosphate-induced delayed neurotoxicity (Abou-Donia, 1981).

Other variables, besides species, must also be considered. One of these is the strain of animal used. For example, it has been demonstrated that rats inbred from the Fischer strain are behaviourally different from Zivic-Miller rats, which are derived from the Sprague Dawley strain (Barrett et al., 1973; Ray & Barrett, 1975). Rats of the Fischer strain rapidly learn both where and when to run in a discriminated Y-maze avoidance task, whereas Sprague Dawley rats eventually learn where to escape but not when to avoid shock. The administration of amphetamine produces a dramatic improvement in the avoidance response of Sprague Dawley rats, whereas little or no behavioural facilitation is observed in the Fischer strain of rat (Barrett et al., 1974). Festing (1979) has reviewed the properties of isogenic and nonisogenic stocks and their relation to toxicity testing.

Since an environmental agent may have a selective effect on either the male or female, gender cannot be ignored when assessing neurotoxicity. For example, sex differences have been seen for the toxic effects of polychlorinated hydrocarbons (Lamartiniere et al., 1979); gonadal hormones influence the biotransformation and toxicity of DDT (Durham et al., 1956) and parathion (Agrawal et al., 1982).

Another important factor is the age of the animal. It is well known that the effects of a toxic agent may vary dramatically depending on the stage of maturation of the animal (Damstra & Bondy, 1982; Hunt et al., 1982). For example, it has been established that young animals of otherwise sensitive species are not susceptible to organophosphate-induced delayed neurotoxicity (Abou-Donia, 1981). It has been suggested that, under conditions where exposure may occur pre- or perinatally, animals of both sexes should be tested at all stages of maturation (Spyker, 1975).

Each of these considerations relates to extrapolation, a subject discussed in detail in WHO (1978). Quantitative and qualitative differences in sensitivity to, and body distribution of, chemicals affect extrapolation significantly. A better understanding of structure-activity relationships, pharmacokinetics, and mechanisms of toxicity will facilitate cross-species extrapolation (Dixon, 1976).

relatively nonspecific effects related to inhibition of growth or decreases in food or water consumption. This is particularly true in studies involving developing organisms.

Another variable is the housing conditions of the experimental animal. In some cases, animals are housed individually in home cages during pharmacological or toxicological studies. This arrangement can alter the responsiveness of the subjects to drugs. Pirch & Rech (1968) found that alpha-methyltyrosine, a depletor of brain norepinephrine and dopamine, produced less depression of motor activity and rotorod performance in rats isolated for 34 days than in grouped rats. The potentiating effects of crowding on the toxicity of amphetamine in mice are also well known (Chance, 1946).

It has been well established that numerous biological systems, ranging from metabolic pathways to behaviour of the whole organism, exhibit rhythmic changes in amplitude (Scheving et al., 1974). Classes of behaviour that show circadian rhythms include feeding, drinking, sleeping, motor activity, and mating (Rusak & Zucker, 1975). There is growing literature on how biological rhythms influence the pharmacological and toxicological response to chemicals (Reiter & MacPhail, 1982). These biological rhythms cannot be ignored and must be either controlled for in the study or studied explicitly.

2.2 Statistical Analysis

2.2.1 Type I and Type II errors

All fields of biological research have at least one feature in common: inherent variability in their data. When there is considerable variation in the experimental material and when it is not feasible to examine the entire population, the research worker is forced to give a probability statement concerning any treatment differences observed. In order to do this, it is necessary for the study to be designed in such a way that statistical analysis of the data will yield a valid answer to the question, "What is the likelihood that the differences observed could have occurred by chance?" Thus, a null hypothesis is set up, i.e., a statement that there is no difference between the parameters or the distributions being estimated by the samples. Taking the simplest case (e.g., Student's t-test), the null hypothesis is that there is no difference between the mean values for 2 populations (e.g., control versus treated). When the null hypothesis is accepted, this may be either right or wrong. A Type I error (false positive) is made when the null hypothesis is rejected and is, in fact, true. A Type II error (false negative) is

2.1.4 Dosing regimen

Some compounds produce toxic effects following a single exposure (e.g., trimethyltin, organophosphates); for others, cumulative effects follow prolonged or repeated exposure (e.g., acrylamide). In environmental toxicology, the detection of cumulative toxicity following continued (or intermittent) exposure is a major goal. Thus, a multiple-dosing regimen is most frequently used. It is important to assess the toxicity at various intervals, since both quantitative and qualitative changes in the response to environmental factors can occur on repeated exposure, or even with time following a single exposure (Evans & Weiss, 1978). Assessments should be made for some time following cessation of the dosing regimen, since it is of interest to determine the reversibility of any effects noted during the dosing phase and to note any post-dosing effects.

2.1.5 Functional reserve and adaptation

Functional reserve is the excess capacity possessed by the nervous system. Thus, a portion of the nervous system can be damaged, and this damage can go undetected by the usual functional tests. The situation in which a change in function was observed at one time, but can no longer be detected by the usual functional tests, is referred to as adaptation and presumably reflects compensatory processes.

If a part of a redundant system is damaged, it is reasonable to assume that the reserve potential has been reduced. If compensatory changes have occurred, the ability of a system to make further compensatory changes may also have been reduced. One way to assess such changes is to incorporate in the test procedures one or more conditions in which the system(s) or organism(s) are placed under stress. The combination of the test substance plus stress may result in a greater deficit in performance than can be seen in animals receiving either the stress or the toxicant only. Examples of stressors that have been used are pharmacological changes such as ethanol, muscular or work stress, exposure to cold, or auditory and electrical stimuli (Lehrer, 1974; Pavlenko, 1975); it is expected that other powerful stressors include those referred to as psychological or psychic.

2.1.6 Other factors

Several additional factors should be carefully considered in designing neurotoxicological tests. One condition that may affect toxicity is the nutritional state of the animal. Changes attributed to exposure to toxicants might be due to

(e) recognize the existence of controversies or differences of opinion in any of the above areas (Bennett & Bowers, 1976).

Clearly, it is beyond the scope of this section to discuss these at length. Similarly, it should be clear that to abide by these principles, frequent and close consultation with a biostatistican may be necessary. Moreover, such consultation should occur before the study is conducted, not afterwards. Consulted beforehand, the statistician can give the guidance necessary for the proper design of the study. Once the study is completed, statistical manipulation cannot compensate for an ill-conceived experimental design.

Different statistical techniques are based on different assumptions, either with respect to the nature of the data, their distribution, or both. Also, the power of different techniques differs. In statistics, power refers to the ability of a test to detect the alternative hypothesis (i.e., that there is a difference) when it is true. Given two tests and a particular level of alpha (e.g., $\underline{P}$ = 0.05), the test with the greater power will detect a significant difference with a smaller sample size compared with the test having lesser power, providing that the assumptions underlying the tests are true. Non-parametric alternatives are available in most cases where the assumptions of parametric tests are not valid. Gad & Wiel (1982) present a "statistical testing decision tree" for selecting the most appropriate test based on whether or not the data are quantitative (continuous) or qualitative (discontinuous) in nature and/or normally distributed. Gad (1982) has also examined the statistical tests most commonly used in behavioural toxicology for different types of observations (data) and suggests procedures that are more appropriate.

Although much more could be said about statistics, it is hoped that the above comments will serve as a warning that the prudent investigator should become facile with experimental design and statistics or work together with a biostatistician, or both.

made when the null hypothesis is accepted and is, in fact, false.

The probability of making a Type I error is called alpha and is fixed before the study is carried out. If something is statistically significant at $\underline{P} = 0.05$, this means that the probability that these results could have occurred by chance is 0.05. The inference is that there is a "real" difference, but this can be wrong, and, in fact, there is a one in twenty chance that it is.

There are two characteristics about neurotoxicology that make it highly likely that one or more Type I errors may occur in any given study. These are (a) the use of multiple tests (measuring multiple parameters), and (b) repeated measurements using the same animal in the same test. Multiple tests are used because of the complexity of the nervous system and the need to assess sensory and motor function as well as more complex behaviour such as discrimination and learning processes. Repeated testing is done because changes in the response to agents can occur on repeated exposure, or even with time following a single exposure (Evans & Weiss, 1978). Thus, in any given study, there are a number of statistical tests of hypotheses. The greater the number of statistical tests of hypotheses, the higher the probability of obtaining Type I errors (false positives). Although problems created by multiple comparisons can be dealt with statistically, to a certain extent, it is imperative to look at the internal consistency of the data and not simply at the presence or absence of statistical significance. Nothing, of course, can take the place of a well-designed study with a clear statement of its purpose. In any case, when in doubt, repetition of the study is in order, if it is sufficiently important.

Variable data can increase the probability of a Type II error (false negative). A Type II error is made when the null hypothesis is accepted and is, in fact, false. The probability of making such an error is called Beta. The value of Beta is seldom, if ever, known. Its relative magnitude can be approximated and depends on:

(a) the distance between the population parameters being estimated by the samples (population means in the case of Student's t);

(b) the value selected for alpha (the probability of making a Type I error or rejecting the null hypothesis when it is, in fact, true); and

(c) the sample size.

The smaller the distance between the population parameters, the larger will be beta. Beta varies inversely with alpha, and both decrease as sample size increases. Thus, if the data are highly variable, a large sample size is needed to detect a small effect. In selecting sample size, these factors must be taken into consideration. When the sample size is determined, the size of the difference that is detectable has also been determined. The smaller the sample size, the larger the change has to be in order to be statistically significant. Techniques are available that identify the sample size needed to detect either a given incidence of occurrence (power function) or a given change in magnitude on the basis of an estimate of the variability in the population(s). Their use is strongly urged. Too many studies have been conducted with sample sizes that were not adequate to detect any real but subtle effect. This topic has been discussed in detail by Dews (1982).

Unfortunately, it is not possible to increase the sample size at will. Therefore, other means must be used in an attempt to reveal individual sensitivity to a given toxicant. In addition to statistical analysis, the raw data should be examined (this is always true, regardless of the results). If any trends exist, it may be necessary to repeat the study. Alternatively, the data may be examined for a change in variability, since a common observation of near-threshold doses of environmental toxicants seems to be an increase in the variability of the data (Evans & Weiss, 1978). This increase in variability is a clue that certain individuals in the population are being affected differentially. Moreover, statistical procedures exist for comparing the degree of variability between control and treated groups (e.g., Steel & Torrie, 1960).

2.2.2   Selection of the appropriate statistical test(s)

In the selection of statistical test(s), it is essential for the investigator to:

(a) be able to choose a technique that is appropriate for the data and hypothesis;

(b) understand the assumptions being made when carrying out the statistical test;

(c) be able to execute the procedure correctly;

(d) be able to interpret the results correctly; and

3. TEST METHODS IN BEHAVIOURAL TOXICOLOGY

3.1 Introduction

Behaviour has been used to study the adverse effects of chemical and/or physical agents on intact organisms. Behavioural toxicology draws on the fields of experimental psychology, behavioural pharmacology, and behavioural brain research.

Behavioural toxicology plays an important role within the broader field of neurotoxicology for two reasons. The first is that the behaviour of an organism is important in itself. As mentioned in the introductory chapter, the nervous system (and consequently behaviour) is influenced by the functioning of other organ systems. Thus, regardless of whether the site of action is the nervous system or some other organ system, toxicant-induced changes in performance, sensorimotor function, or cognitive function adversely affect the organism and its ability to interact with its environment. The second reason is that behaviour is the final product of nervous system activity and, therefore, toxicant-induced changes in the nervous system may be reflected by behavioural changes. Thus, behavioural analysis serves as a useful tool for measuring neurotoxicity (i.e., the direct action of a chemical on neural tissue). This approach can be compared to measuring blood flow or cardiac output as an index of cardiovascular toxicity (i.e., the use of functional measures to evaluate the status of a target organ).

This section deals with the use of animal behavioural testing to estimate neurotoxicity in human beings. It should be noted that Citovic (1930), a student of Pavlov, reported the use of conditioned reflexes to study the neurotoxic effects of gasoline and acetone. Soviet and Eastern European toxicologists have commonly incorporated behavioural testing in their studies. However, scientists in Canada, western Europe, and the USA placed heavy emphasis in chemical toxicity studies on defining pathological changes following exposure, and it was not until 1969 that the Annual Review of Pharmacology in the USA included a section on behavioural toxicology (Weiss & Laties, 1969). Since then, behavioural toxicology has been the subject of numerous books, symposia, and reviews (Anger & Johnson, 1985). Thus, it is a relatively new discipline, and its specific methodology continues to evolve rapidly. In this section, the major emphasis is placed on the basic principles of behavioural toxicity testing. General approaches are discussed in relation to their use in a comprehensive test strategy for evaluating behavioural toxicity. As discussed later, any such strategy should include tests that adequately evaluate each of the 5 main functional categories listed in Table 1 (p. 17). Strengths and weaknesses of existing methods are also considered, together with future methodological directions and needs.

3.2 Classes of Behaviour

In the experimental analysis of behaviour, the primary focus is on defining the functional relationships between an organism's behaviour and its environment, i.e., in this context, everything that has an effect on the organism. Behaviour is a dynamic process, since it reflects changes in the interaction of an organism with its environment. Thus, an important feature of behavioural toxicology is that the effects of a toxic agent may depend largely on environmental circumstances. In other words, with a given toxic effect on the nervous system, the observed behavioural effects may (and probably will) depend on environmental factors.

The basic units of behaviour are termed responses. Aspects of the external or internal environment that affect behaviour are termed stimuli. Behavioural responses have been typically divided into two classes based on the functional relations that control their occurrence. One class of behaviour is controlled mainly or exclusively by the prior occurrence of an event (stimulus) in the environment. Such responses are referred to as elicited or respondent behaviour. The events are called eliciting stimuli, and the responses are called respondents. The other class of behaviour is controlled mainly or exclusively by its consequences and is referred to as operant or emitted behaviour. Behaviour may be either unconditioned (unlearned) or conditioned (learned). Conditioning refers to the modification of a response that results from an organism's interaction with its environment. In general, however, when a response is said to have been conditioned, this usually implies that the conditioning was done explicitly as part of an experimental procedure rather than as a result of some other experience the organism encountered.

Descriptions of conditioning as either "operant" or "respondent" can be confusing, in that behaviour is also characterized by these terms. The issue becomes clearer if it is realized that operant and respondent conditioning are operationally defined procedures of behavioural modification, whereas operant and respondent responses are descriptions of two classes of behaviours, both of which are modifiable through conditioning.

3.2.1 Respondent behaviour

Respondent behaviours are those that are reliably elicited by a specific observable stimulus. Two major features of a respondent behaviour are: (a) its occurrence depends on the frequency of occurrence of the eliciting stimulus; and (b) its consequences do not affect its frequency, or affects it only to a minor extent.

Respondents frequently take the form of simple or complex reflexes and typically involve smooth muscles, glandular secretion, autonomic responses, or environmentally-elicited effector responses. Examples are the auditory startle response (Hoffman & Fleshler, 1963), olfactory responses, such as homing behaviour (Gregory & Pfaff, 1971), visually guided responses, such as optokinetic nystagmus (King & Vestal, 1974), and responses elicited by somaesthetic cues, such as negative geotaxis (Alder & Zbinden, 1977).

Respondent behaviour can be quantified in a number of ways, including: (a) latency of the response from onset of the stimulus; (b) stimulus intensity required to elicit the response (threshold); and (c) magnitude of the response. Response magnitude can be measured either directly (e.g., force, duration) or by the use of rating scales (Irwin, 1968). A respondent generally occurs in close temporal contiguity with its eliciting stimulus, and its occurrence is independent of stimulus parameters such as duration, intensity, and frequency.

Various types of respondent behaviour, both unconditioned and conditioned, have been used in behavioural toxicology (Irwin, 1968; Pavlenko, 1975). Several features of unconditioned respondent behaviour argue for its use. Perhaps the most important features are that: (a) stimulus-response relations are well defined and easily controlled; and (b) such methods require no prior training of the animal and, therefore, are easily and rapidly administered.

The use of unconditioned respondent behaviour has generally been focused on 2 response classes:

(a) reflexes, in which the response is limited to a specific effector system, such as skeletal muscle (motor response) or smooth muscle (autonomic response); and

(b) taxis, in which the whole animal orients itself towards or away from a particular stimulus.

Reflexes have been more extensively studied. An example is the acoustic startle response, which occurs following an intense auditory stimulus. A principle motor component of this response-forelimb extension can be readily measured. The acoustic startle response has been used widely in the study of drugs (Davis, 1980) and more recently in the study of other neurotoxic substances (Reiter et al., 1980; Squibb & Tilson, 1982).

Unconditioned respondent behaviour has also found specific application in the study of effects of toxic substances on the developing nervous system. Developmental profiles for many types of unconditioned respondent behaviour have been well described for the rat (Altman & Sudarshan, 1975) and mouse (Fox, 1965). Because normal development of these responses is very closely timed, measurements of their developmental time-course have been widely used as an index of nervous system development. A number of investigators have used measurement of this behaviour as an index of toxicity (Rodier, 1978; Butcher & Vorhees, 1979).

Respondent behaviour can also be conditioned using the classical techniques initially described by Pavlov (1927). This involves the pairing of a previously neutral stimulus (one that does not normally elicit a response) with an eliciting stimulus. Through repeated pairings, the neutral (conditioned) stimulus comes to elicit a conditioned response. Respondent conditioning is illustrated in the following example: when food (unconditioned stimulus) is placed in a dog's mouth, it elicits salivation (unconditioned response). If a tone (conditioned stimulus) is sounded just before food is placed in the dog's mouth, the tone itself eventually comes to elicit salivation (conditioned response) in the absence of food presentation. Although a variety of different controlling stimuli can be used in classical conditioning, responses are limited to those for which there is an initial unconditioned eliciting stimulus. The conditioned response can be quantified in terms of its latency, magnitude, and frequency of occurrence. If the conditioned stimulus occurs repeatedly in the absence of the unconditioned stimulus, the conditioned response becomes progressively weaker and eventually disappears; this process is called extinction.

Since movement is the basic measurement of behaviour, the majority of conditioned reflex procedures evaluate motor responses. The acquisition of a conditioned response can be studied by gradually producing it. This requires careful control over external conditions, particularly the intensity and timing of both the conditioned and unconditioned stimuli. Since the rate of acquisition of a conditioned response depends on the functional status of the nervous system, such procedures are useful in the study of behavioural toxicity.

Pavlenko (1975) reviewed the extensive use of conditioning by behavioural toxicologists in the USSR. Classical conditioning methods were divided into 2 groups. The first group, "defence-motor reflexes", generally involved a motor response to an electrical stimulation applied to the skin. The second group, "alimentary-motor reflexes", generally involved the response of a hungry animal to the presentation of food. Soviet investigators have frequently studied the rate of acquisition of such conditioned responses in the presence of toxic substances. According to Pavlenko (1975), small dosages of toxic agents more readily affect the acquisition of conditioned responses than the performance of firmly established conditioned responses (Shandala et al., 1980).

3.2.2 Operant behaviour

Behaviour that appears to occur in the absence of an eliciting stimulus is referred to as an emitted or operant response. Operant responses are movements of the organism that operate on (or change) the environment. Although these responses may occur in the presence of many environmental stimuli, they are not readily associated with an identifiable eliciting stimulus, and their occurrence is controlled mainly by their consequences. However, some responses are known to include both respondent and operant components. The best-known example is provided by bird pecks, which are controlled partly by eliciting stimuli and partly by response consequences, apparently in relation to their consummatory and non-consummatory functions, respectively.

Emitted behaviour generally occurs with a close temporal relationship to the deprivation and presentation of particular environmental conditions, regardless of whether the deprivation produces an obvious physiological change. For example, an animal given access to a novel environment will show a characteristic temporal pattern of "exploratory" activity, with initial high levels of activity diminishing to low levels. Availability of the novel environment is associated with motor activity, but the novel environment is not an eliciting stimulus. Under these conditions, operant behaviour can be studied by observing all or part of the animal's behaviour during a specified period of time.

Various rating scales have been used to quantify the frequency of occurrence and/or magnitude of selected operant responses (Irwin, 1968). A more detailed approach has been to quantify the frequency, duration, and temporal patterning of selected emitted responses using time-lapse photographic analysis (Norton, 1973).

Operant or instrumental conditioning refers to the modification of an operant behaviour by the control of its consequences. The following example illustrates operant conditioning: a food-deprived rat is placed in a chamber equipped with a food dispenser and with a lever projecting from a wall. If depression of the lever is followed by presentation of food, there is an increased likelihood that this response (lever press) will occur again. That is, the consequences of behaviour (e.g., receipt of food) come to control the occurrence of the response (pressing the lever).

In contrast to classical conditioning, in operant conditioning, mere temporal contiguity between stimulus events is not sufficient for learning to take place and it is the consequences of behaviour that control the learning process. This concept was first introduced by Thorndike (1932) in his "Law of Effect," which dealt with the nature of events that can control operant behaviour. When the occurrence of an event following a response increases the probability that the response will occur again, the event is termed a reinforcing stimulus or reinforcer. The presentation of the reinforcing stimulus is termed reinforcement. Events that serve as reinforcers when presented (e.g., food) are termed positive reinforcers; events that reinforce when terminated (e.g., electric shock) are termed negative reinforcers. If, on the other hand, the probability of occurrence of a response is decreased by its consequences, the consequences are termed punishment. An operant is defined as the properties of behaviour upon which reinforcement (or punishment) is contingent. In the previous example, for instance, pressing the lever is the operant. There are, of course, many ways that the rat can press the lever during operant conditioning. Nevertheless, each press is considered to belong to a single response class: the operant.

Some response outputs, such as the bird pecks mentioned above, can be modified by experience as a function both of stimulus-response contingencies (so-called autoshaping) and response-reinforcement contingencies. In other words, both classical and operant conditioning can contribute to the changes observed in a particular response output, and this may have to be taken into account when assessing treatment effects.

One of the strong features of operant conditioning is the broad range of behaviour that can be controlled and the new responses that can be generated. In practice, the responses most commonly selected for study meet four basic criteria: (a) they are easily identified and readily counted; (b) they are easily recorded with automated equipment; (c) their emission requires little time; and (d) they are readily repeatable (Kelleher & Morse, 1968).

Reinforcement need not accompany every response in order to maintain that response. More commonly, reinforcement occurs intermittently and according to a schedule defining a sequential and/or temporal relationship between the response and its reinforcement. Schedules of reinforcement are of critical importance in determining both an organism's rate and pattern of responding, and the effects of a chemical (Kelleher & Morse, 1968). Different schedules of reinforcement have been shown to generate characteristic patterns of behaviour between species, even when using a wide variety of response topographies and reinforcing stimuli. Through the systematic development of schedules of reinforcement (Ferster & Skinner, 1957), operant conditioning has become an important tool in behavioural pharmacology and, more recently, in behavioural toxicology (Laties, 1982).

3.3 Test Methods

3.3.1 General attributes of behavioural methods

Behavioural toxicity test methods vary in sensitivity, specificity, validity, replicability, and cost. These factors, in combination with the "question(s) to be asked" at a particular stage of testing, will strongly influence the choice of method. It is also important to take into account the extent to which the results of such tests may be applicable to human beings.

3.3.1.1 Sensitivity and specificity

Sensitivity refers to the ability of a test method to detect the occurrence of a toxicant-induced behavioural change. If the objective of a study is to detect whether a chemical produces behavioural toxicity, a test with moderate sensitivity may be sufficient, particularly when there is no limitation on dose range. However, if the intention is to define threshold levels of exposure associated with behavioural effects, sensitivity becomes extremely important.

Specificity has been used in several contexts. In one, it refers to the ability to give a negative finding when no behavioural effect has occurred. In another, it refers to the number of nervous system functions it reflects. Some tests are relatively specific. Many are of limited specificity in that they reflect changes in a number of nervous system functions (which, in turn, may reflect changes in other organ systems). In this context, specificity is interrelated with validity (section 3.3.1.2). Since behavioural tests rely on motor performance, all lack specificity to a certain extent.

3.3.1.2 Validity

Validity is concerned with whether a chemically-induced change in a behavioural response reflects only the change(s) in the behaviour to be measured. If, for example, a test is used to assess learning, the possibility must be considered that factors other than learning (e.g., motivational levels, motor function) may influence the test results. Some understanding of test validity is essential for the proper interpretation of behavioural toxicity test results. The use of a variety of behavioural tests, thereby determining a behavioural profile, can be useful in establishing the validity of a particular test.

3.3.1.3 Replicability

Replicability refers to the ability of a test method to give consistent results in repeated studies (both within and across laboratories); it is somewhat analogous to precision. Precise protocols and strict attention to experimental detail will lessen variability and, therefore, increase replicability.

3.3.1.4 Costs

The costs of performing different types of behavioural analyses will have some influence on test selection. During the early stages of testing, when the focus is on detecting the presence of behavioural toxicity, cost will considerably influence the choice of method. It is unreasonable to use a highly sophisticated procedure requiring expensive equipment to detect whether a compound has potential behavioural toxicity whenever a cheaper alternative is available. In contrast, studies to determine the no-observed-adverse-effect levels of a chemical may justify the use of expensive, time-consuming methods.

3.3.2 Primary tests

Tests can be divided into primary and secondary categories. Primary tests are used for screening neurotoxicity, but such tests must forecast the potential of such chemicals to produce effects. Secondary tests are used to further characterize the nature of these effects. Since many functions are mediated by unique neural substrates and many chemicals produce rather selective effects, it is important to employ a variety of tests that measure different behavioural functions.

3.3.2.1 Functional observation battery

Functional observation batteries are designed to detect major overt neurotoxic effects. A number of investigators have proposed series of tests that are generally intended to evaluate various aspects of behavioural, neurological, and autonomic status (Irwin, 1968; Pavlenko, 1975; Pryor et al., 1983). These batteries consist of series of semiquantitative measurements appropriate for the initial level of behavioural assessment (e.g., tremor, convulsions, ataxia, autonomic signs, paralysis). The tests are, in effect, rating scales concerning the presence or absence (and, in some cases, the relative degree of presence) of certain reflexes. In addition, eating and drinking behaviour and body weight should also be considered in the context of primary behavioural assessment.

The major advantages of these tests are that they can be easily administered and can provide some indication of the possible functional alterations produced by exposure. Potential problems include insufficient interobserver reliability, difficulty in defining certain measures (e.g., stupor), and the tendency towards subjective bias. As a consequence, it is essential that observations be carried out by individuals who are blind to the groups.

Many types of screening tests are currently used to assess the effects of neurotoxic agents on motor and reflex function. The simplest of these include observational assessments of body posture, muscle tone, equilibrium and gait, and righting reflexes (Irwin, 1968; Snyder & Braun, 1977). These tests are quantal or categorical at best, and are generally subjective. Larger animals permit a conventional neurological examination similar to that used with human beings (Abou-Donia et al., 1983).

3.3.2.2 Motor activity

Spontaneous motor activity in rodents has been extensively used in behavioural toxicology (Reiter, 1978; Reiter & MacPhail, 1979). Movement within the living space or environment is a high-probability response in animals and can be easily manipulated by environmental changes, including exposure to neurotoxic agents. Although seemingly simple, locomotor activity is very complex behaviour comprising a variety of motor acts, such as horizontally- and vertically-directed movement, sniffing, and grooming. Rating scales have been developed to fractionate locomotor activity into its relative components (Draper, 1967). The measures used most often in behavioural toxicology are horizontally- and vertically-directed activity (Reiter & MacPhail, 1979). A large variety of devices, automated and nonautomated, have been invented to measure motor activity. Following exposure to a neurotoxic agent, various qualitative and quantitative changes can be observed, depending on the apparatus that is used. For example, the figure-eight maze has been used extensively and successfully to detect effects produced by a number of chemicals (Reiter, 1983).

Although the figure-eight maze has been used as a residential maze to measure toxic effects on diurnal activity patterns, recent research has almost exclusively employed shorter time intervals (Reiter, 1983). Elsner et al. (1979) have reported a method for the continuous monitoring of spontaneous locomotor patterns in rats. Using computer-assisted techniques, these investigators found that methylmercury treatment lowered activity during the night portion of the diurnal cycle.

The complexity of motor activity is emphasized by the finding that low-level exposure to volatile organic solvents increases activity, whereas high level exposure decreases it (Horvath & Frantik, 1973). Positive results in a motor activity test usually require further testing to identify the precise function affected. Activity is not a unitary measure and a change in the frequency of this behaviour can reflect toxicant-induced changes in one or more sensory or motor functions, alterations in reactivity (excitability) or motivational states, or perturbations of a variety of regulatory states (e.g., diurnal cycles, energy balance of the animal). For example, a decrease in activity might mean that the animal is paralysed or, perhaps, that it suffers from "general malaise". Thus, if a change in motor activity is observed, additional tests are needed to determine the cause.

3.3.3 Secondary tests

3.3.3.1 Intermittent schedules of reinforcement

Performance generated by intermittent schedules of reinforcement (Ferster & Skinner, 1957; Reynolds, 1958; Kelleher & Morse, 1968; Schoenfeld, 1970) has played an important role in behavioural pharmacology and is proving a useful tool in behavioural toxicology (Laties, 1982).

Most intermittent schedules involve reinforcement as a function of the number of responses emitted, some temporal requirements for emission of responses, or both. Ratio schedules require the animal to emit a fixed number of responses (fixed ratio or FR) or a number distributed around some average (variable ratio or VR) in order to be reinforced. As the ratio requirement is increased, the latency of the first response increases; however, once responding begins, it typically proceeds at a high and constant rate. Interval schedules require that a certain length of time should elapse before the response is reinforced. This may be a fixed time (fixed interval or FI) or time distributed around an average (variable interval, VI). Although only one response need be emitted at the end of the interval to cause reinforcement, the organism typically emits many responses during the interval. Interval schedules usually generate lower rates of responding than ratio schedules. The FI schedule generates a characteristic pattern of responding for which a variety of parameters potentially sensitive to disruption by neurotoxic agents can be analysed (Kelleher & Morse, 1968). Other commonly-used intermittent schedules specify the temporal spacing of responses. In the differential reinforcement of low rate (DRL) schedule, the organism is required to wait a specific time between responses in order to be reinforced. In the differential reinforcement of high rate (DRH) schedule, the organism is required to emit a specified number of responses within a specified (short) time, and thus responds at a high rate.

Intermittent schedules of reinforcement can be combined to form more complicated "multiple" schedules of reinforcement. A classic example is the combination of FR and FI schedules presented in succession during a single test session; the resulting multiple schedule is termed a multiple FR-FI schedule. Each component of the multiple schedule is independent and occurs in the presence of a different external discriminative stimulus, which signals it. The schedule components are typically presented in alternating fashion, allowing the investigator to collect data on both types of behaviour almost simultaneously. Individual schedule components can be combined in other ways with different levels of complexity (Tilson & Harry, 1982). Such schedules are not yet in general use in behavioural toxicology.

The most common measure of performance with intermittent schedules is response rate (responses per unit time). This measure may be sufficient to establish whether there is an effect in a particular schedule or schedule component before grossly toxic levels are reached. A measure that may be more sensitive to the effects of toxic agents is the inter-response time (IRT) distribution (Schoenfeld, 1970). For example, IRT distribution was a sensitive indicator of lead toxicity in rats performing on a multiple FI-FR schedule (Angell & Weiss, 1982).

Another measure that may be a sensitive indicator of behavioural toxicity is variability in performance, both within and across sessions (Schoenfeld, 1970). Near the no-observed-adverse-effect level, variability between animals may be increased in the exposed group(s); variablity between groups may be a sensitive indicator of toxicity. For example, Laties (1982) studied the effects of methylmercury exposure in the pigeon using a fixed consecutive number (FCN) procedure, in which the animal was required to respond on one key a specified number of times consecutively before responding on another key to be reinforced. Methylmercury exposure decreased the mean number of times pigeons responded on the first key before switching (run length) and increased the standard deviation of the run length within a session. Rice (in press) found increases in both within- and between-session variability in FI response rate in monkeys exposed developmentally to lead at doses insufficient to produce changes in rate.

Marked differences in individual susceptibility to the effects of lead exposure on development have been observed using FI performance in the rat (Cory-Slechta & Thompson, 1979) and monkey (Rice et al., 1979). In general, lower doses increased, and higher doses decreased, the response rate. In the monkey, the IRT distribution remained different between treated and control groups, even though changes in rate disappeared after about 40 min. Remarkable differences in individual susceptibility were also observed on a response duration schedule (Cory-Slechta et al., 1981). In this schedule, the animal was required to depress a lever for a specified time (several seconds) before releasing it. Some of the exposed animals gave performances indistinguishable from those of the controls, while others performed much more poorly than controls. Differences in individual susceptibility may be a common phenomenon, particularly in behavioural toxicology, and should be considered in the determination of no-observed-adverse-effect levels (Dews & Wenger, 1979). An increase in group variability may signal the presence of toxicity in some portion of the population of responders (Good, 1979).

Simple schedules, such as FR, FI, VI, DRL, and continuous avoidance, have been used to detect effects produced by a number of industrial and environmental toxic agents (Padich & Zenick, 1977; Dietz et al., 1978; Geller et al., 1979; Zenick et al., 1979; Leander & MacPhail, 1980; Alfano & Petit, 1981; McMillan, 1982). Perinatal lead exposure resulting in a relatively low body burden of lead produced effects in a DRH schedule in the absence of changes in motor activity (Gross-Selbeck & Gross-Selbeck, 1981).

Multiple schedules offer the opportunity to study behaviour controlled by different variables, which may be differentially sensitive to the effects of toxic agents (this is known to be true for pharmacological agents). For example, toluene decreased the response rate in the FR component and increased the rate in the DRL component of a multiple schedule (Colotla et al., 1979); furthermore, the relative sensitivities of the two components were different. The multiple FI-FR schedule has proved particularly useful in detecting behavioural toxicity (Levine, 1976; Dews & Wenger, 1979; Leander & MacPhail, 1980; Angell & Weiss, 1982; McMillan, 1982).

Intermittent schedules of reinforcement can be used to monitor effects other than, or in addition to, direct effects on the central nervous system. These may include damage to the peripheral nervous system or to some other organ system that results in general malaise (Laties, 1982). For example, acrylamide, an organic solvent that produces a "dying back" axonopathy, produced decreases in FR response rate (Tilson et al., 1980). The schedules typically produce high response rates and thus may be sensitive to impairment in motor function. Exposure to ozone resulted in decreased responding on an FI schedule; this was interpreted as resulting from general discomfort produced by ozone (Weiss et al., 1981).

In addition to schedules that maintain behaviour by positive reinforcement, responding can be maintained by negative reinforcement. Avoidance schedules are either continuous (i.e., each response postpones shock by a fixed amount of time) or discrete-trial (each shock is preceded by a warning signal during which a response will prevent punishment). Avoidance schedules have been used extensively in the study of anticholinesterase compounds, including pesticides, in order to assess dose-response relationships, the time course of behavioural depression during acute intoxication, and the effects of repeated exposure (Bignami et al., 1975). Their usefulness in the assessment of treatment effects is shown in the extensive drug literature. In fact, the confounding of treatment effects with "motivational" changes is postulated to be less of a problem with avoidance tasks than with appetitive tasks (positive reinforcement). Furthermore, once acquired, avoidance responses can be maintained at fairly stable levels without the precautions necessary in the study of appetitive responses (e.g., daily control of food or fluid intake and/or body weight), though induction of stress responses and changes in pain sensitivity must be considered.

3.3.3.2 Motor function

A variety of techniques developed to evaluate motor function have been used; these include performance on a rotating rod or treadmill (Frantik, 1970), swimming to exhaustion (Bhagat & Wheeler, 1973), or suspension from a horizontal rod (Molinengo & Orsetti, 1976). One increasingly used technique is the quantification of hindlimb splay. Edwards & Parker (1977) inked the feet of rats, dropped the animals from a specified height, and measured the distance between the digit marks. Schallert et al. (1978) used a similar technique of inking paws to evaluate abnormal gait in rats treated centrally with 6-hydroxydopamine.

A negative geotaxis procedure was used by Pryor et al. (1983) to evaluate neurotoxic agent-induced alteration in motor coordination. Reduction in grip strength is a frequently reported neurological sign in human beings; fore-

and hindlimb grip strength in rats and mice has been quantified using commercially available strain gauges (Meyer et al., 1979).

Tremor is a common neurotoxic effect. A number of rating scales and semiquantitative procedures to measure tremor are available (Gerhart et al., 1982). A simple but expensive spectral analysis technique that permits rapid evaluation of tremor in freely moving animals has been reported by Gerhart et al. (1982).

Other more complicated techniques have been devised to measure motor deficits in laboratory animals. For example, Falk (1970) trained animals to press a lever within a designated range of force for a given period. Falk and others (Fowler & Price, 1978) used this procedure to study the effects of toxic agents on fine motor control.

3.3.3.3 Sensory function

Exposure to toxic chemicals can cause a wide range of sensory effects. Alterations in sensory processes, such as paraesthesia or visual or auditory impairment, are frequently among the first signs of toxicity in human beings exposed to toxic agents (Damstra, 1978). In animals, "psychophysical" methods are used to arrive at some estimation of differential response in the presence of a stimulus varied across some physical dimension (Stebbins, 1970). The great majority of psychophysical studies have been carried out on non-human primates and birds; ideally, such studies should be conducted on species in which sensory function closely resembles that of human beings. Psychophysical methods range from those that assess a gross loss of sensation to those that provide a sensitive and precise analysis of changes in threshold levels and other ancillary or complex sensory phenomena.

One of the least complex approaches to the study of sensory deficits is based on the localization or orientation response. Marshall and colleagues (Marshall & Teitelbaum, 1974; Marshall et al., 1974; Marshall, 1975) have described a battery of observational tests in which a visual, auditory, olfactory, or dermal stimulus is delivered to the organism. The presence or absence of a localization or orientation response to the source of this stimulus is then recorded. Such techniques have been used to demonstrate sensory inattention as well as hyperexcitability in rats having lesions in various regions of the brain. Pavlenko (1975) has described a variety of stimulus-elicited orientation reflexes used in the USSR. Despite the fact that observational tests are simple to perform, they are labour intensive, especially if the necessary inter-rater reliability scales are used. However, the scoring of the tests is frequently subjective and necessitates testing under "blind conditions." Finally, the data are usually quantal (i.e., the response is scored as either present or absent) or categorical (scored on a rating scale). Thus, interpretation of the results is difficult, particularly in repeated-measure designs.

Several attempts have been made to develop simple yet objective tests for sensory dysfunction in rodents. Some investigators have used measurement of the acoustic startle reflex (i.e., measurement of the presence (and magnitude) or absence of response to a novel sound or tone) as a screen for auditory dysfunction. Pain sensitivity can be assessed using standard psychopharmacological techniques measuring reaction times to a noxious stimulus (Pryor et al., 1983). Electrical stimulation of the tooth pulp is a sensitive method to detect change in pain sensitivity (Costa & Murad, 1969). The flinch-jump technique also is used extensively to determine changes in pain threshold (Evans, 1962). Taste reactivity has been assessed using taste aversion procedures (Kodama et al., 1978). Depth perception has been assessed using a visual cliff procedure, which measures whether or not an animal chooses to step onto a nearby platform or floor ("shallow" floor) in preference to one that may be perceived as more distant ("deep" floor) (Sloane et al., 1978). Another simple test of visual function is the optokinetic drum, which relies on the optokinetic nystagmus or optomotor response (i.e., tracking a moving object with the eyes and head for a certain distance until the head is repositioned back into the frontal plane). On the basis of this measure, a procedure was developed that was believed to assess visual acuity as well as colour vision (Wallman, 1975).

Changes in reflex response have been monitored in a variety of ways. The ability of a stimulus to inhibit a reflex response has been used to detect changes in auditory threshold in the rat (Young & Fechter, 1983). Reflex responses (e.g., front-paw withdrawal or ear flexion) following electric shock have been used extensively in the USSR to determine changes in pain threshold or detection of electromagnetic fields (Speranskij, 1965).

More complicated paradigms have been used to assess sensory dysfunction in more precise ways. Mazes and maze-like apparatus appear to have some use for evaluating certain sensory deficits (e.g., visual or somesthetic) in rats (Overmann, 1977; Post et al., 1973). However, as Evans (1978) pointed out, the relative contributions of motor and higher-level functions should be carefully distinguished when interpreting results of such studies.

Some of the more precise methods for evaluating subtle sensory deficits involve operant techniques. In these studies, a response (e.g., pressing a lever) is maintained by food or electric shock. Once the animal has learned to make the response only under certain stimulus conditions, the intensity of the stimulus can be varied and the response determined as a function of the intensity. Such techniques have been used to show auditory loss following exposure to kanamycin (Harpur & d'Arcy, 1975; Chiba & Ando, 1976). Merigan (1979) used reinforcement of the identification of spots of light by a monkey with a fixed gaze to demonstrate the presence of scotomas following methylmercury exposure.

Olfactory (Wood, 1978), shock or pain (Weiss & Laties, 1961), and vibration (Maurissen, 1979) thresholds have been determined using operant techniques. Operant methods also have been used to study the effects of toxic exposure on more complex sensory phenomena, including light flicker discrimination (Schechter & Winter, 1971), critical flicker frequency (Merigan, 1979), and discrimination of the duration of a visual or auditory stimulus (Johnson et al., 1975).

Chemical agents can act as reinforcing and internal discriminative stimuli and gain control of a variety of behavioural responses. In fact, Wood (1979) demonstrated the abuse potential of toluene in an operant paradigm analogous to drug self-administration.

Pryor et al. (1983) reported on the use of a relatively simple psychophysical technique to assess 3 sensory modalities concurrently in the same animal. In this procedure, rats learned to climb or pull a rope to avoid a noxious electric footshock. Eventually, the response was brought under the control of three conditioned stimuli: a tone, a low-intensity, nonaversive current on the floor, and a change in intensity of the chamber house light. Various intensities of each stimulus were presented, permitting generation of a quasipsychophysical response function. Once the animals were trained, they were exposed to toxic agents and the changes in responding were measured.

Another procedure that shows promise in the assessment of sensory function is the use of prepulse inhibition of the acoustic startle reflex. By varying the intensity of the prepulse stimulus, treatment effects on sensory acuity can be assessed. Such a procedure has been used to study the effects of triethyltin on auditory functions in experimental animals (Young & Fechter, 1983).

3.3.3.4 Cognitive function

Within general psychology, "cognition" refers to the processes by which knowledge of surroundings is gained; perception, thinking, learning, and memory refer to different aspects of cognitive processes. The attribute "cognitive" has been extended by analogy to classify animal behaviour, as well. Tolman (1948) used the concept of "cognitive maps" to account for the fact that rats are able to acquire and retain information about spatial relationships in experimental mazes, and to use this "latent" information for subsequent learning. Another example of the study of cognitive processes in animals are the "insight" studies on chimpanzees (Kohler, 1976), in which behaviour resembling human problem-solving has been demonstrated. Thus, cognitive functions cover a much broader field than just approach-avoidance learning (the prevailing paradigm in today's behavioural toxicology). In practice, however, learning and memory are the cognitive functions that have received particular attention in animal studies, because they are amenable to quantification and because the abilities to learn and to remember have obvious adaptive value for an organism. The capacity to learn permits an organism to escape or avoid situations, approach desirable objects, and store these contingencies for future use.

Behavioural toxicologists have used a variety of experimental paradigms to assess learning and memory in laboratory animals. A few procedures have been developed to measure the ability to adjust to a new contingency once an initial task has been learned. Studies have involved conditioned respondent as well as conditioned operant behaviours.

(a) Procedures using negative reinforcement

In passive avoidance techniques, the animal is trained to withhold a response, to avoid punishment. A standard procedure is to put the animal on the lighted side of a shuttle box and to shock it as it enters the dark compartment (Wolf, 1976). After a given interval of time, the animal is returned to the apparatus and is given no shock. Dependent variables include the initial response latency, subsequent response latencies, number of positive responses, number of compartment crossings, and total time spent in either compartment on retesting for a fixed interval of time. Walsh et al. (1982b) used one-way passive avoidance to demonstrate trimethyl tin-induced memory deficits in adult rats in the absence of changes in sensitivity to shock. This technique was used to demonstrate learning/memory deficit in rats exposed neonatally to chlordecone (Mactutus et al., 1982).

Passive avoidance techniques have the advantages of speed, ease of performance, and low cost. They have the disadvantage of producing highly variable results if performed under inadequate test conditions or if the appropriate retention intervals are not used. Finally, it is imperative that the nonassociative variables mentioned above be measured and that alterations in motivational factors (e.g., changes in "pain thresholds" to footshock) be evaluated.

One-way active avoidance tasks require the animal to respond in order to escape or avoid negative reinforcement. Typically, an animal is placed in one compartment of a shuttle box, where it can be shocked. Once the active avoidance or escape response to the neighbouring compartment has been registered, the animal is returned to the original compartment and the process is repeated. Using this type of test, Tilson et al. (1979a) reported that rats with long-term exposure to chlordecone learned to avoid as rapidly as controls but displayed a marked retention deficit when retested several days later.

Another variant of the shock-motivated learning task is the two-way shuttle box paradigm. In this procedure, rats learn to shuttle from one compartment to another in the presence of a warning signal in order to escape or avoid electric footshock. Unlike one-way avoidance, the animals must learn to return to a compartment where they have just been shocked. Interesting differences in effects can be observed between one- and two-way procedures. For example, Sobotka et al. (1975) reported that rats exposed neonatally to lead performed as well as controls in a one-way shock avoidance test but displayed significant deficits in a two-way paradigm.

In general, one- and two-way avoidance tasks entail one training trial or several discrete massed training trials. These are followed by one or more trials in which retention is assessed. Dependent variables for both types of avoidance tasks are avoidance latencies, number of correct responses, and number of trials to a predetermined criterion of learning. A useful measure of activity is number of inter-trial crossings; this information can aid in interpretation of treatment effects. Tilson et al. (1982a) reported a triethyl lead-induced facilitation of two-way shuttle-box performance that was not associated with altered motor activity (inter-trial crossings) or flinch-jump threshold.

The symmetrical Y maze is a somewhat more complete learning task than either one- or two-way avoidance. In this procedure, a light or tone is activated in one of two arms of a maze not occupied by the animal. The animal is given a predetermined amount of time to run to the proper arm to avoid electric shock. Dependent variables include all those previously mentioned for avoidance procedures as well as number of correct choices. The Y maze has been used very successfully by Vorhees (1974) to study learning ability in rats exposed in utero to vitamin A. The paradigm involves two types of learning: when to run and where to run. These may be affected differently by treatment (Ray & Barrett, 1975).

As pointed out in section 2, strain differences must also be considered: rats of the Fischer strain easily learn when and where to avoid, but Sprague Dawley rats do not readily learn when to avoid (Tilson & Harry, 1982).

Experimental paradigms that involve other tasks and types of negative reinforcement have been used to assess learning. In the water maze, animals are placed in a maze filled with water and are required to learn a series of correct turns in order to gain access to an exit ramp. Learning trials are preceded by straight-channel swimming trials as an adaptive procedure and to determine if there are any measurable neuromotor deficits. Frequently, initial learning is tested in 6 trials on day 1, retention is tested after 7 days, and then reversal-learning is tested by changing the position of the escape ramp. Performance measures are swimming time, number of errors, and number of correct choices. Water maze studies have revealed learning deficits in animals exposed developmentally to vitamin A (Vorhees et al., 1978) and to lead or mercury (Brady et al., 1976; Zenick et al., 1979). Vergieva & Zaikov (1981) studied the performance in a water maze of adult rats after short- and long-term inhalation of styrene.

(b) Procedures using positive reinforcement

Learning and memory can also be assessed in paradigms that use positive reinforcement. A number of techniques involve positive reinforcement of discrimination tasks. The type of discrimination can be spatial or sensory (visual, auditory). Spatial discrimination tasks usually involve simple T mazes or more complicated versions of the T maze, such as the Hebb-Williams maze, which actually is a sequence of successive T mazes. Dependent measures are the number of correct trials or the time needed to reach the goalbox. Snowdon (1973) found that rats exposed to lead neonatally showed impaired performance in a Hebb-Williams maze, whereas rats exposed postweaning or as adults did not.

Visual discrimination tasks frequently take the form of simultaneous two-choice pattern discrimination. Dependent variables usually are the number of correct discriminations or number of trials needed to reach a predetermined criterion. Winneke et al. (1977) trained food-deprived rats to make a discrimination based on either the size (circle size) or orientation (horizontal versus vertical stripes) of a cue placed on a door in a maze leading to food reinforcement. Lead-exposed animals took longer to acquire the more difficult size discrimination but resembled controls in learning the orientation-cued response. Since visual deficit, as assessed by visual evoked potentials, did not occur until blood-lead levels exceeded 400 µg/litre (Winneke, 1979), visual dysfunction could be ruled out as an alternative explanation for the lead-induced learning deficit, which occurred at blood-lead levels below 200 µg/litre (Winneke et al., 1983).

In a similar two-choice visual discrimination task (Tilson et al., 1982b), animals were trained to make a nose-poke response to the side of a cue panel that contained a visual cue. After an animal had learned the correct discrimination (which occurred over a period of days), the contingency was reversed, i.e., a response to the side in which the cue lamp remained unlit was reinforced. Rats exposed to chlordecone during development showed a trend towards altered acquisition performance and were markedly different in the way that they responded during the reversal phase of this test.

Visual discrimination learning has also been used to study the effects on monkeys of lead exposure during the developmental period (Bushnell & Bowman, 1979; Rice & Willes, 1979). In these studies, lead-induced deficit was observed only in the more demanding discrimination reversal paradigm. This constitutes evidence for "silent" toxicities that become apparent only with tasks of increased complexity. Similar conclusions can be drawn from studies on rats in which lead-induced learning deficit was demonstrated for difficult but not simple discrimination tasks (Winneke et al., 1977, 1983).

The previous measures of learning have involved between-subject designs that can require large numbers of animals, if there is large inter-animal variability. A within-subject design enables the effects of chemical agents to be evaluated with reference to the animal's stable pre-exposure baseline and so controls for inter-animal variablilty. One such paradigm is repeated chain acquisition: a animal is given a series of 4 buttons that must be pressed in a specific order. The order is changed each day, so that a new but generally similar repeatable task is presented to the animal each day. In this paradigm, carbaryl affected the rate of performance of monkeys, but errors were not as clearly affected (Anger & Setyes, 1979). A similar method was used to detect alteration of response patterning by lead (Dietz et al., 1978) and mercuric chloride (Leander et al., 1977). In addition to studies of the effects of chemical agents on the acquisition of new behaviour, there have been studies of memory, and the persistence or lack of persistence of acquired information with the passage of time. Memory has been studied using between-subject designs employing a radial maze.

The radial-arm maze (RAM) is a complex spatial learning task in which animals must "remember" a list of previously entered and unentered feeders during a free-choice test session (Olton el al., 1979, 1980). The RAM is believed to be useful in studying working (information relevant to a single trial), as well as reference memory (information relevant to all trials). The most commonly used RAM consists of a circular arena from which eight equidistant arms radiate like spokes from a wheel. A trial begins with all arms baited and ends when all pellets have been consumed or when a fixed period of time has elapsed. The most effective strategy for solving the maze is to enter and eat in each of the arms only once. Results can be expressed in several ways such as: (a) number of correct choices in the first eight selections (control rats will often obtain all eight pellets without an error); (b) total number of errors made in obtaining the eight pellets. Walsh et al. (1982b) reported that trimethyltin-exposed rats displayed impaired performance in this task and that the behavioural deficit might be due to an alteration in the integrity of limbic forebrain structures such as the hippocampus. The RAM has also been used to study loss of spatial memory as a function of isolation in darkness and of time elapsed since initial learning (Buresova & Bures, 1982).

Memory has been studied using operant discrete trial techniques, which enable greater control over the stimuli applied in this study and thus more sensitivity, but require more training. Animals are trained to respond in a series of trials that are separated by time intervals. Performance in a trial depends on information presented in the previous trial. These operant techniques always use within-subject designs and have proved useful in the study of drugs because they make it possible to dissociate the effects on memory from the effects on motivation or motor control. For example, it has been shown that scopolamine impairs memory but does not interfere with responding in delayed, go-no go, alternation (Heise & Milar, 1984). This technique was applied in behavioural toxicology using delayed, spatial alternation, which combined two toxicologically sensitive tasks, discrimination and reversal spatial memory (Heise, 1983). It was found that carbaryl decreased both memory and responding.

Modifications of Harlow's "learning set formation paradigm" for use with primates also deserves mention in this context. In this task, the animal is given a great number of discrimination problems to be solved successively. As training progresses, new problems are solved faster and faster (i.e., the number of trials necessary to solve each problem decreases with increasing number of problems). Lilienthal et al. (1983) used this task to demonstrate lead-induced cognitive deficit in rhesus monkeys; simple discrimination learning was not affected, but transfer of learning was. Thus, acquisition of information was not impaired but memory for previously acquired information was disrupted.

3.3.3.5 Eating and drinking behaviour

Many of the behavioural tests described above use food as the primary reinforcer to get the animal to perform an instrumental response. Eating is thus involved in the results of the various tests employed. However, eating can also be used in the assessment of the potential behavioural toxicity of chemical compounds. Eating and drinking are naturally occurring behaviour that can be measured in the animals' laboratory environment; once a stable eating and drinking pattern is established, toxic agents can be introduced and the resulting alteration in behaviour measured (Tilson & Cabe, 1978). For example, since it has been shown that carbon monoxide and hypoxia depress food intake, Annau (1975) compared the effects of both conditions on food and water intake in naive rats. Two control groups were compared with groups exposed to 250, 500, and 1000 ppm carbon monoxide and 16%, 14%, and 10% oxygen. Although both experimental conditions produced a decrease in body weight and in food and water intake, the shapes of the resulting curves were very different, suggesting that carbon monoxide may not act on these biological systems in an identical manner to hypoxia; in fact, it appears that hypoxia has a more severe effect on behaviour than the equivalent concentration of carbon monoxide. A more recent investigation (Bloom et al., 1983) showed that subconvulsive doses of pyrethroid insecticides reduced variable interval performance as well as food intake, indicating that further attention should be devoted to the relationship between eating and drinking and other behavioural response changes.

Eating responses in rodents also altered when a food having a specific taste was paired with an illness produced either by irradiation or by the administration of a toxic substance, thus making it possible to assess the aversive properties of the agent tested. This conditioned taste aversion has been employed as an experimental preparation in the evaluation of the unconditioned stimulus functions of several toxic substances, such as chlordimeform (MacPhail & Leander, 1982), trialkyltin (MacPhail, 1982), and industrial solvents (Vila & Colotla, 1981).

Schedule-induced, or adjunctive, drinking is another type of consummatory behaviour (Colotla, 1981) of interest to the neurobehavioural toxicologist for two reasons: first, it has been demonstrated that the procedure can generate "voluntary" consumption of alcohol and several other drugs, and second, it produces a consistent and regular post-reinforcement behaviour pattern that is sensitive to the effects of several drugs (Colota, 1981). Although, to date, no reports have appeared in the neurotoxicological literature on the effects of toxic substances on adjunctive behaviour, this type of eating response may be useful as part of a test battery for neurobehavioural toxicity.

3.3.3.6 Social behaviour

Social behaviour implies behaviour involving two or more individuals (Hinde, 1974), which means that almost all activities of an animal are, or can be, social. Since social behaviour represents a complex set of interactions, its investigation in the laboratory is not simple: each behavioural response of an animal living in a group (including a pair) may be influenced by previous interactions with members of the group and by the behavioural characteristics of individuals forming the group.

Although considerable literature exists on the social behaviour of laboratory animals, additional methodological development is necessary before it can be included in routine toxicological evaluations. Methodological and theoretical problems include the definition of individual classes of social behaviour, and the generalization of results obtained with different species. There are problems dealing with the objectivity of measurement, standardization of testing procedure, and statistical evaluation. Use of laboratory animals (mice, rats) raises the question of adequacy of the social environment created by the research worker because the laboratory environment is very different from the social environment of the species in the wild.

Although social behaviour has not been used extensively in toxicology, it has found some use as a diagnostic tool in psychopharmacology, where various kinds of social interaction have differentiated between the effects of drugs of different pharmacological classes (Miczek & Barry, 1976). This body of psychopharmacological work demonstrates that the behavioural effects of different chemicals can be modified by the social environment and thus can differ from the effects in isolated animals.

Two basic approaches have been used to study social behaviour in animals. The first evaluates the impact of social setting on the various types of behaviour in animals living for long periods in semi-natural or artificial conditions. Under this test situation, housing conditions and population density can be shown to affect various behavioural and physiological responses. Litter size, for example, was shown to influence an animal's response to various stimuli; the effect depended not only on nutritional status but also on social behaviour (Frankova, 1970). Overcrowding has been shown to affect behaviour, as well as endocrine and other organ systems functions (Thiessen, 1964). Chemicals such as amphetamine

have greater toxicity when administered to grouped mice
(Chance, 1946). There are differences between individually-
and colony-housed rats in the oral ingestion of morphine
(Alexander et al., 1981), aversiveness to Naloxone (Pilcher &
Jones, 1981), and ethanol consumption (Kulkosky et al., 1980).

A second more common approach to the study of social
behaviour is the short-term observation of an animal's
behavioural response to another individual (e.g., cage mate,
sexual partner) or group. Here the pair or group is observed
out of the home cage, usually in a specially equipped box.
Various chemically-induced disruptions of different social
interactions have been reported for rodents and primates.
Silverman (1965) developed criteria for paired interactions in
rats (e.g., mating aggression, submission, escape) and
demonstrated the effects of drugs on these categories of
social behaviour. Various other studies (Frankova, 1977;
Krsiak, 1979; File, 1980) have evaluated effects of drugs on
isolated and group-bound mice and rats. Cutler (1977) demonstrated that lead exposure disrupts social behaviour in mice.

Other studies have investigated the effects of chemicals
on the social behaviour of non-human primates. Apfelbach &
Delgado (1974) administered chlordiazepoxide to gibbon colo-
nies and observed a decrease in mobility and aggressive acts
and increased play, grooming, and water intake. Bushnell &
Bowman (1979) showed that long-term lead ingestion affected
play and other social behaviour in infant rhesus monkeys.

The types of social behaviour most frequently examined for
effects of chemicals (especially drugs) are dominance and
submission (Baenninger, 1966), isolation-induced aggression
(Krsiak, 1979; Eichelman et al., 1981), sexual behaviour, and
maternal behaviour (Grota & Ader, 1969; Frankova, 1971, 1977).

3.3.4 Strengths and weaknesses of various methods

Many of the test methods described in this section have
been used successfully to model human neurotoxicity, while the
relationship of findings of other tests to human disease is
not known. Also, of course, each method or group of methods
has its proponents; often the individuals or groups who have
developed and used it extensively. However, over the past
decade, there has been a broadening in the exchange of test
methods between research laboratories and countries. Some
obvious examples are the use in the USSR of T-maze and
shuttle-box avoidance testing (Kholodov & Solov'eva 1971;
Asabayev et al., 1972) and of unique test devices for teaching
simple discrimination using positive reinforcement
(Kotliarevski, 1957; Masterov, 1974; Medvedev, 1975); the use
in Eastern Europe and South America of operant techniques

(Colotla et al., 1979; Vergieva & Zaikov, 1981); and the use in the USA and South America of reflex conditioning to elucidate pharmacological and toxicological effects (Costa & Murad, 1969; Young & Fechter, 1983).

It is probably true that investigators who have perfected the technical aspects of their own paradigms "get the most out of them." Behavioural science, as any other science, involves a set of techniques of such sophistication that many are best learned in the laboratories in which they were developed. This presents some difficulties in inter-country transfer of methods and the unrestrained endorsement of methods developed in another country with other behavioural/psychological traditions. Those who adopt a method for which they have no ready contacts with experienced investigators may abandon it as "insensitive", when the only problem may be technical errors in application.

Respondent behaviours have the advantage of being rapidly formed. In most cases, only 40 - 60 trials or tests in a single day are required for their formation, and the behaviours may be elicited periodically during long-term exposure studies with no diminution in their usefulness. Pure muscle responses or integrated motor activity (as in a shuttle box or startle response chamber) can be measured. These methods can reflect both increases (stimulation) and decreases (depression) in responding, and can be completely automated, thus eliminating subjective factors.

Operant methods can entail the kinds of complex behaviour needed to evaluate such complex factors as learning. Their proponents also point out that they can be used to measure fundamental behavioural properties related to the control of behaviour. However, operant paradigms require several weeks for the animals to reach stability on a schedule of reinforcement and a great deal of time of a highly skilled research worker to train animals to perform complex tasks. As with respondent methods, operant methods can detect both increases and decreases in responding and can be completely automated.

In addition, it is axiomatic that behaviour is essentially an integration of sensory, cognitive, and motor processes. The specificity of a toxic effect on any behavioural parameters must always be evaluated in the context of the experimental design and in conjunction with controls for effects on the other systems.

3.4 Research Needs

3.4.1 Compensatory mechanisms

Because the functional redundancy of the nervous system can mask some perturbations, procedures need to be devised and used that will reveal toxic effects that are not apparent under normal test conditions. Challenges by environmental and pharmacological agents have proved to be useful in the search for subclinical toxic effects, and their use is recommended. By creating additional demands on behavioural integration, challenges can reveal "hidden" functional deficits (Hughes & Sparber, 1978; Tilson et al., 1979b; Tilson & Squibb, 1982). The pharmacological challenges most commonly used are psychoactive drugs and substances that mimic or block the actions of putative neurotransmitters or alter their synthesis, storage, or release. Some common stresses that have been used as environmental challenges are alterations in circadian rhythms, density of housing, noise level, and ambient temperature (MacPhail et al., 1983). Studies to increase the understanding of subclinical toxic effects and provide information concerning appropriate rationale for the selection of specific challenges represent an important research need (Tilson & Mitchell, 1984).

Adaptive changes in the nervous system can also occur after repeated exposures to high levels of a toxic agent. There is an initial decrement or increment in behaviour after the first exposure, but then there is a recovery of function to the preexposure levels as exposure continues. This apparent return to normal function results from adaptive changes in the systems that control behaviour. Sometimes this change is due to tolerance within the affected systems, but in other cases, there could be a redundant system that enables the return to the pre-exposure state. Research on these forms of compensatory mechanisms is to be encouraged.

3.4.2 Method development and refinement

Development of methods, evaluation, and refinement remain basic needs in behavioural toxicology. Many behavioural test strategies and test batteries have been proposed for the longitudinal assessment of behavioural function in animals exposed to toxic agents either during development or as adults (Butcher, 1976; Grant, 1976; Rodier, 1978; Buelke-Sam & Kimmel, 1979; Butcher & Vorhees, 1979; Tilson et al., 1979c; Zbinden, 1981; Mitchell et al., 1982; Vorhees & Butcher, 1982). Most authors agree that it is essential that a core of functions should be assessed, since it is unlikely that any single one will be sensitive to all toxic agents. The guidelines for reproductive testing in France, Japan, and the United Kingdom require assessment of several functions but do not specify exact tests. Many fear premature standardization of specific tests while behavioural toxicology is still in its initial period of growth (Weiss & Laties, 1979). Development, validation, and standardization of primary (screening) tests need to continue and could be facilitated by the use of reference compounds (Horvath & Frantik, 1973).

An easily obtained source of information that deserves more attention, especially in long-term studies, is the uninterrupted behaviour of animals in their home cages. Food and water intake can provide information on homeostatic functioning, while a measure of activity can assess changes in movement patterns or in the circadian rhythm of activity.

There does not yet appear to be an animal model of fatigue. Further elaboration of animal models to evaluate fatigue dissociated from motivational factors needs consideration.

It is generally accepted that complex tasks are more sensitive to chemical disruption than simple tasks, and that a behaviour that is not fully learned or practiced is more sensitive to chemical disruption than one that is well learned and established. These and many related assumptions require testing. Publication of skillfully selected comparative data from a variety of laboratories will assist all investigators in the future selection of test methods. In particular, more and better methods involving complex tasks that may be relatable to human beings are required.

Increased and improved automation of test methods is another need. Automation can eliminate observer (and even trainer) bias, and should be pursued where feasible. The increasing availability of inexpensive microprocessors continues to put more and more laboratories in a position to acquire the central tool for automation of more complex methods.

4. NEUROPHYSIOLOGICAL METHODS IN NEUROTOXICOLOGY

4.1 Introduction

The term neurophysiology may refer to all studies of the function of the nervous system. As such, it could include studies of conditioning and behaviour as well as electrical recordings obtained from the nervous sytem. However, for the purposes of this section, a more restricted definition of neurophysiology will be used, with few exceptions, to mean the study, by measurement of electrical activity, of nervous system activity.

Even with this restricted definition, an enormous array of neurophysiological methods is available to the neurotoxicologist. Depending on the methods selected, neurophysiological studies can be used to achieve goals as diverse as detecting neurotoxicity, characterizing neurotoxicity (i.e., which neural systems are involved) and unravelling mechanisms of neurotoxicity. Each of the methods selected for presentation below can be used to achieve at least one of these goals. In addition, some of the methods can be used in human studies as well as those on laboratory animals, thereby providing ready opportunity for cross-species extrapolation.

While the use of physiological methods to assess the impact of toxic chemicals on the nervous system has a long history (Citovich, 1930; Zakusov, 1936), the development of more sophisticated recording devices has led to an expansion of their use. As the technology to use these techniques develops, it becomes progressively more affordable, and should therefore become even more popular in the near future.

In this section, the neurophysiological evaluation of neurotoxicity will be discussed in terms of assessment of the peripheral nervous system, the autonomic nervous system, and the central nervous system. With careful reading of the different sections, it should become evident that some methods described in one place may be useful under other circumstances. In the final section, a few issues pertaining to the interpretation of neurophysiological data will be addressed.

4.2 Methods for Evaluation of the Peripheral Nervous System

4.2.1 Conduction velocity

Many substances are known to produce alterations in the peripheral nervous system (Spencer & Schaumburg, 1980), and evaluation of the functional integrity of peripheral nerves is the subject of the clinical science known as electrodiagnosis (Johnson, B.L., 1980). Conduction velocity, the speed at which action potentials are conducted along axons and nerves, is the most widely used measure of peripheral nerve function. Conduction velocity is usually measured in such a way that the activity of the fastest conducting axons is assessed. Changes in conduction velocity that occur following exposure to toxic substances producing axonopathy are reliable, but usually not large, often ranging from 10 to 30% of control values (Gilliatt, 1973). On the other hand, demyelination produces large decrements (50%) in conduction velocity (McDonald, 1963).

Principles involved in performing conduction velocity studies have been presented by Daube (1980), and techniques using rodents have been described, in detail, by others; some of these toxicological studies have been reviewed by Johnson, B.L. (1980) and Fox et al. (1982).

Many other techniques besides conduction velocity have been applied in the assessment of peripheral nerve function. They include assessment of the refractory period (Hopf & Eysholdt, 1978; Lowitzsch et al., 1981), assessment of the extent to which axons and nerves can follow trains of stimuli occurring at high rates (Lehmann & Tachmann, 1974), accommmodation indices (Quevedo et al., 1980), and the use of collision techniques for selectively blocking activity of some nerve axons to study others (Kimura, 1976). Some of these techniques will certainly provide even greater sensitivity than the simple velocity measurements in common use.

4.2.2 Peripheral nerve terminal function

Methods for evaluating function in peripheral sensory receptors are particularly valuable in neurotoxicology. Toxic agents that exhibit a preference for the distal ends of long peripheral nerves, a dying-back neuropathy, or distal axonopathy might be expected to alter or impair the sensory function of these receptors (Fox et al., 1982). Indeed, in the case of proprioceptors, such as muscle spindles, neurotoxic insult can contribute to ataxia, areflexia, and incoordination (Lowndes et al., 1978a,b). Detailed discussion of the methods can be found in Fox et al. (1982). Although measuring peripheral nerve terminal function is more difficult than measuring peripheral nerve conduction velocity, such measurements are important since alteration of function in the terminal portions of axons frequently precedes alterations in conduction velocity. For example, function of muscle spindles (Lowndes et al, 1978a,b), motor nerve terminals (Lowndes & Baker 1976), and primary afferent terminals (Goldstein et al., 1981) has been reported to be compromised by toxic agents, long before any alterations are detectable in conduction parameters. Another advantage of these techniques is that, not only can the presence of neurotoxicity be detected, but the site(s) of neurotoxic action can also be investigated.

4.2.3 Electromyography (EMG)

The recording of biopotentials from muscle (electromyography) has been extensively used in human clinical studies in the diagnosis of certain diseases of the muscle (Johnson, E.W., 1980). EMG is an objective and sensitive method for the detection of changes in neuromuscular function. Altered neuromuscular function using EMG was detected in organophosphorus insecticide workers who did not exhibit other detectable signs and symptoms of poisoning including depressed blood cholinesterase activity (Drenth et al., 1972; Roberts, 1977).

EMG methods have been litle used for the study of neurotoxic substances in experimental animals. According to Johnson, B.L. (1980), there are probably two reasons for this. First, few toxicologists are trained in EMG procedures. Second, one important component of an EMG examination involves the evaluation of the voluntary graded contraction of the muscles. This is sometimes difficult to control in experimental animals. Nevertheless, methods using experimental animals are available (Johnson, B.L., 1980), and have been used successfully to study the neurotoxic effects of methyl n-butyl ketone (Mendell et al., 1974) and manganese (Ulrich et al., 1979).

Electromyography is used to study direct toxic effects on muscles. Evoked muscle responses to nerve stimulation are invaluable in examining the neuromuscular junction, which can be affected by various neurotoxic agents (e.g., botulinum and tetanus toxins and organophosphate insecticides).

4.2.4 Spinal reflex excitablility

Segmental spinal monosynaptic and polysynaptic reflexes are relatively simple functions of the central nervous system that can be easily evaluated by quantitative techniques (Mikiskova & Mikiska, 1968; Fox et al., 1982). Many of the methods used in animals are direct laboratory counterparts of some of the clinically used neurological tests in human beings. There are two basic approaches. One does not requires any invasive procedures and thus is most akin to the tests used in human beings. The other involves electrophysiological techniques for examining the effects of neurotoxic agents on mono- and polysynaptic reflexes.

In the non-invasive techniques, the functional state of the reflex arch is inferred either from the latency and size of the reflex response evoked by stimuli of a predetermined intensity (Zakusov, 1953) or from the stimulus intensity (threshold) just sufficient to elicit a detectable response (Mikiskova & Mikiska, 1968). The threshold approach has been used by Mikiskova & Mikiska (1966, 1968) to study a variety of volatile solvents. In their view, the procedure is useful both as a screening test and in estimating the relative toxicities of substances. It is critical that a stimulator with a constant current output is used so that the stimulating current does not depend on the resistance of the skin and electrodes.

The time required for a stimulus to a peripheral nerve to reach the spinal cord and return to the site of stimulation directly (F response), particularly after crossing a single synapse (H response), can indicate the excitability of the motoneuron pool. Fox et al. (1982) present electrophysiological techniques for examining the effects of neurotoxic agents on mono- and polysynaptic reflexes. This approach can provide better clues than the non-invasive approach concerning possible site(s) of action for the neurotoxic agent, but is considerably more time consuming. Moreover, the manner in which it is generally carried out (decerebrate animals) precludes repeated testing on the same animal. Thus, for most types of investigations (screening, determining threshold concentrations for effect) the non-invasive approach is preferable.

4.3 Methods for Evaluation of the Autonomic Nervous System

Compared to other approaches, relatively little effort has been expended in assessing the impact of suspected toxic agents on the activity of the autonomic nervous system. Most neurophysiological methods are designed to measure relatively rapid events, and therefore they are not particularly well suited to the evaluation of the autonomic nervous system. However, a few exceptions are noteworthy.

4.3.1 Electrocardiography (EKG)

Electrocardiography supplements other neurophysiological methods by providing data on the central and peripheral nervous control of autonomic functions. However, the interpretation of EKG changes is complex and must take into account direct effects on the myocardium (Mikiskova & Mikiska, 1968).

4.3.2 Blood pressure

Concomitant recording of EKG and blood pressure using environmental and pharmacological challenges is an approach worthy of consideration for evaluating animals exposed to suspected toxic agents. Altered circulatory responses to these types of stimuli may yield important information concerning the functional status of the autonomic nervous system. Indeed, exaggerated responses to vasopressor and cardiac acceleratory stimuli would suggest that such exposure might be accompanied by a higher risk of cardiovascular disease.

4.4 Methods for Evaluation of the Central Nervous System

4.4.1 Spontaneous activity - electroencephalography (EEG)

EEG analysis was one of the first forms of electro-diagnosis of nervous system dysfunction. Since its discovery by Berger (1929), there have been progressively more sophisticated attempts at analysis, and progressively greater promises for its value. At present, the EEG is used widely in clinical settings, and consequently a variety of sources are available describing the technical details of recording, analysis, and interpretation (Basar, 1980; Niedermeyer & Lopes da Silva, 1982). In clinical neurology, the EEG has been used for the diagnosis and description of epilepsy, localization of tumours, description of sleep stage, as well as many other neurological disorders (Niedermeyer & Lopes da Silva, 1982). It has been used less often for the detection of subtle toxic agent-induced dysfunction, though it is an integral part of Soviet and Eastern European neurotoxicological studies (Horvath & Frantik, 1973, 1976).

The normal EEG, whether recorded from the scalp or with indwelling electrodes in specific brain regions, has an amplitude of up to about 100 uv. The useful frequency spectrum of the EEG is below 50 Hz, though higher frequencies are encountered in certain brain regions (Johnson, B.L., 1980). It is common to analyse the scalp-recorded EEG according to the amount of electrical activity contained within specific frequency bands, specifically: δ (2 - 4 Hz), θ (4 - 8 Hz), α (8 - 13 Hz), β_1 (13 - 20), and β_2 (20 - 30 Hz) (Lindsley & Wicke, 1974). A variety of electronic frequency analysers, as well as computer procedures, are available for use in analysing the power spectrum of the EEG throughout the entire frequency range or within selected frequency bands (Lindsley & Wicke, 1974).

When electrodes are implanted in specific brain areas, the resultant EEG can be used to assess the effects of toxicants on these different brain areas or structures. Also, specific brain regions (e.g., the hippocampus) have particular patterns of after-discharge following chemical or electrical stimulation, which can be quantitatively examined and used as a tool in neurotoxicology (Dyer et al., 1979).

It should be pointed out, however, that disassociation between the EEG pattern and behaviour can occur. For example, high voltage-slow activity (generally associated with sleep) has been seen following administration of atropine in animals that seemed to be excited (Bradley, 1958). Also, low voltage-fast activity (generally associated with arousal or with REM sleep) has been reported following physostigmine in animals that seemed to be asleep (Bradley, 1958). Thus, caution must be used in the interpretation of EEG changes alone.

Extensive discussions and references, concerning the use of the EEG in neurotoxicology, are presented in Horvath & Michalova (1956), Mikiskova & Mikiska (1968), Johnson, B.L. (1980), and Fox et al. (1982). The full potential of this technique in neurotoxicology has not yet been fully exploited. However, it is clear that modern electronic and computer facilities are required to maximize its use. Moreover, changes in the pattern of the EEG elicited by stimuli producing arousal (light, sound, electrical stimulation) (Desi & Sos, 1962; 1963) or produced by sleep (Fodor, et al., 1973) will most probably enhance its usefulness in neurotoxicology (Zilov et al., 1983). It should be noted that changes in the EEG have been reported after treatment with organophosphate compounds before depression of acetylcholinesterase activity was noted in the blood or brain tissue (Desi et al., 1974). In a more recent study, Desi (1983) compared changes in EEG with a behavioural test (maze), cholinesterase enzyme activity, and several general toxicological tests following exposure to 13 different pesticides. He concluded that the EEG was the most sensitive test for the detection of early and mild changes caused by these pesticides.

4.4.2 Sensory systems

In studies of sensory systems, the response of the nervous system to a well defined, yet physiological, input stimulus can be evaluated. Precise specification and control of the input stimulus reduces variability in the measured end-points, and increases the clarity with which toxicant-induced alterations are detected. Certain neurotoxic agents seem to have a particular affinity for sensory systems (e.g., methanol). Furthermore, there are few cases when toxicant-induced damage to a non-sensory system is not parallelled by damage in sensory systems.

The overall functional integrity of a sensory system is most directly assessed using evoked potential techniques. These techniques require the application of a discrete sensory stimulus, and averaging of the electrical activity from an appropriate neural pathway or brain area during a brief (e.g., 0.3 second) post stimulus epoch over repeated (e.g., 100) trials. Such averaging reveals a characteristic waveform that is specific to a particular modality, stimulus, electrode location, or species. Alterations in the latency from the stimulus to the specific peaks in the waveform, or in the amplitude of specific peaks in the waveform, are diagnostic of dysfunction.

Sensory-evoked potential techniques are widely used in neurological clinics (Beck et al., 1975), and are becoming increasingly used in neurotoxicity evaluations. Since they may be readily recorded from unanaesthetized unrestrained animals, sensory evoked potentials may be obtained during, and correlated with, behavioural studies. They may detect, with various levels of sensitivity, alterations resulting from exposure to such chemicals as organometals (Dyer et al., 1978) and pesticides (Boyes et al., 1985). More detailed description of the rationale, methods, interpretation, strengths and limitations of sensory evoked potential techniques can be found in Dyer (1985a,b).

4.4.3 General excitablity

A common readily observed consequence of exposure to high concentrations of neurotoxic agents is an alteration in behavioural arousal. While some compounds produce sleep and coma, others produce seizures (Holmstedt, 1959; Lipp, 1968; Joy et al., 1980; Joy, 1982). These alterations may be presumed to reflect disordered excitability of the brain, and have led to the assumption that quantitative measures of excitability would be useful for the detection of dysfunction in this dimension. Four main approaches have been taken in the assessment of general excitability: (a) convulsive phenomena; (b) stimulation of motor cortex; (c) recovery functions; and (d) EEG recordings. EEG recordings have already been discussed in section 4.4.1.

4.4.3.1 Convulsive phenomena

While there are many experimental models of epilepsy (Purpura et al., 1972), not all of these are suitable for the detection and characterization of neurotoxicity. In neurotoxicology, seizure susceptibility has been most often assessed using either electrical stimulation or systemically administered drugs to produce seizures.

Pharmacological stimulation, using agents such as pentylenetetrazol (Metrazol), is simple, quick, and cheap. While interpretation may be complicated if the toxic agent under study alters the metabolism of the convulsant agent, practice has failed to reveal many such instances. Depending on the convulsant selected, the integrity of selected neurochemical systems may be assessed. For example, picrotoxin is presumed to act by blocking activity in GABA-ergic systems.

Electrically induced seizures have been widely used in neurotoxicology. Horvath & Frantik (1979) and Frantik & Benes (1984) evaluated the effects and relative potentials of a wide variety of organic solvents on the extensor phase of electrically induced seizures in rats. They compared the severity of these seizures with other behavioural effects obtained in both laboratory animals and man, thus providing a comparative measure of the relative toxicity of these chemicals. The seizures were suppressed by relatively low air concentrations of most of the solvents tested and this occurred in a concentration-dependent manner.

Electrically-induced after discharges offer the opportunity to study seizure activity in specific brain regions with implanted electrodes in the absence of behavioural correlates. These tests have been used particularly in areas of the limbic system known to be sensitive to neurotoxic agents and to have low seizure thresholds (Dyer et al., 1979).

Repeated elicitation of after-discharges from certain brain regions leads to the progressive recruitment of behavioural correlates by a process known as kindling. The development of kindling-induced seizures, while more time consuming than other methods, may provide more detailed information regarding the nature of alterations produced by the toxic agent. A discussion of kindling as a model for the study of neurotoxic agents can be found in Joy (1985).

4.4.3.2 Stimulation of the cerebral motor cortex

The motor area of the cerebral cortex is preferred because stimulation results in constant, clearly defined motor responses. The procedure is discussed in detail by Benesova et al. (1956), Mikiska (1960), and Mikiskova & Mikiska (1968). Basically, "excitability" is determined by measuring the current required to evoke minimal movement of the contralateral fore limb. Studies can be conducted acutely or with the long-term implantation in animals of electrodes (generally fine screws) touching the motor cortex. Depressant agents uniformly raise the threshold to electrical stimulation (by as much as several fold) whereas stimulant type agents lower it (but to a lesser extent). Effects of drugs and toxic agents in this procedure are cited by Mikiska (1960) and Mikiskova & Mikiska (1968). It should be noted that direct electrical stimulation of central nervous tissues has far more complex consequences than stimulation of peripheral nerve. The stimulus excites thousands of neurons mutually connected by excitatory and inhibitory synapses, which often form reverberating circuits (Mikiskova & Mikiska, 1968). Thus, interpretation concerning the possible mechanism of effect is difficult.

4.4.4.3 Recovery functions

Repeated stimulations may alter the threshold for evoking a response. Neuronal recovery processes are among several neurophysiological challenges reviewed for their relevance for the detection and characterization of neurotoxicity by Dyer & Boyes (1983). While these methods have only recently been used in neurotoxicology, there are a number of instances in which they detect neurotoxic effects earlier than other methods (Dyer & Boyes, 1983).

4.4.4 Cognitive function

Not all evoked potentials are directly related to eliciting sensory stimuli. Parts of some waveforms (most often the "late" or "slow" components) are presumed to be elicited by events that are internal, and may reflect cognitive activity or initiation of motor activity (Otto, 1978). In human beings, changes in one such potential have been associated with extremely low body burdens of lead (Otto et al., 1981). Unambiguous interpretation of such findings is not yet possible, and the methods have not been applied extensively to animal studies. However, increased research activity in this area should make assessing the value of these "slow potentials" more straightforward.

4.4.5 Synaptic and membrane activity

Using appropriate microelectrode neurophysiological techniques, it is possible to determine in a direct way whether exposure to a toxic agent impairs the response properties, synaptic function, or membrane properties of neurons (Fadeev & Andrianov, 1971; Andrianov et al., 1977; Fadeev, 1980; Barker & McKelvy, 1983; Dingledine, 1984). While exquisite in the precision of the information they provide, these techniques are technically difficult and expensive to use, and are most profitably used to assess mechanism of toxicity. Data and discussion of the value of these techniques can be found in Joy (1982), Narahashi (1982), and Narahashi & Haas (1967, 1968); all of these reports consider the effects of organochlorine insecticides and pyrethroid insecticides on properties of neuronal membranes.

4.5 Interpretation Issues

Most neurophysiological methods provide information at several different levels. For purposes of organization, it is convenient to divide the brain into discrete functional systems such as the somatosensory system, the visual system, the extrapyramidal system, etc. While these systems are clearly interrelated, they are almost always treated separately. Most such systems are constructed of neurons with similar membrane and axonal properties, but they differ with respect to their connections, neurotransmitters, and metabolic activity. Thus, evaluation of any one system provides a combination of information, some unique to the system, and some common to most or all neural systems.

The choice of the appropriate neurophysiological methods for a given study depends on the questions posed. If emphasis is on identification of systems involved in the toxicity produced by a specific compound, then gross measures of the functional activity of whole systems are desirable (e.g., evoked potentials in the visual system). On the other hand, if a compound is known to be toxic for a particular system, for example the hippocampus, and the emphasis is on the mechanism of toxicity, then microelectrode techniques may be appropriate. Investigators about to perform neurophysiological studies of neurotoxicity should become familiar with the strengths and limitations of the methods mentioned in this review before selecting one. Furthermore, attention should be paid to the possibility that the toxicant-induced alterations observed reflect secondary dysfunction, which in turn is produced by primary dysfunction in another system. For example, a compound that produces hypothalamic dysfunction and compromises the body's ability to thermo-regulate will appear to produce changes in other systems that are really secondary to hypothermia.

A major advantage of many of the neurophysiological techniques mentioned above (EEG and evoked potential) is that they are readily recorded in human beings as well as laboratory animals. This feature provides a ready framework for cross species extrapolation of data, though considerable work must still be performed before the health implications of alterations in some of these end-points is fully understood. A second important feature is that the relationships between behavioural and electrophysiological alterations produced by toxic agents can be observed in awake subjects, as can any dissociation between these two types of end-points.

Finally, it cannot be emphasized too strongly that the CNS is constantly receiving afferent input and sending efferent output to all the organs of the body. This principle of self-regulation of physiological functions, incorporating the cybernetic principle of feedback gave rise to the functional system theory of Anokhin (1935). This theory has been described in detail by Anokhin (1968, 1974) and Sudakov (1982). According to this theory, functional systems are dynamic self-regulated organizations, the components of which contribute to the attainment of a useful adaptive result for an organism. The components of any given functional system are united or integrated by the afferent and efferent CNS influences impinging on it. The importance of this theory to toxicologists lies in its focus on: (a) adaptive mechanisms; and (b) the inseparable nature between the CNS and the other organs via the afferent input and efferent outflow. First, it is the interference with adaptive mechanisms that gives rise to the signs and symptoms produced by a toxic agent. Second, the inseparable nature of the CNS and other organs complicates localization of the primary target of a toxic agent. Thus, the electrophysiological changes seen in the CNS or the alteration in behaviour may not be due to a primary effect on the CNS, but may rather be the result of alterations in afferent input due to disturbances in peripheral systems such as the gastrointestinal tract, liver, or kidney. Or, the chemical could interfere with a metabolic process common to a number of "functional systems" subserving different biological needs. The lesson, as stated previously in both sections 2 and 3, is that neurotoxicologists must not be too hasty in concluding that any effect observed is due to a direct effect on the CNS. They should, in fact, demonstrate that it is not due to an effect on another organ.

4.6 Summary and Conclusions

Neurophysiological methods are important in animal neurotoxicology. They provide direct laboratory counterparts for many of the tests used in human beings. They can give insight into possible site(s) and mechanism(s) of actions. They can be particularly useful when used concomitantly with behavioural methods. The use of evocative techniques (arousal, stimuli, work loads, interactions with psychopharmacological agents) can increase the sensitivity of the tests for detecting toxicant effects. As with behavioural methods, it is incumbent on the investigator to determine whether an effect on the CNS is due to a primary action of the toxic agent or a secondary one as a result of damage to some other organ, thus altering the afferent input into the CNS or its processing within the CNS.

The most useful techniques for screening are those that are minimally invasive, relatively cheap and rapid to perform, and test neural function in a broad sense. Depending on the particular application, these may include evoked potential, EEG, EMG, excitability, or conduction velocity studies. More restricted use of these techniques, or use of microelectrode techniques, may be useful for further characterizing the systems affected and the mechanisms of action of neurotoxic agents. In some instances, neurophysiological techniques have been reported to be more sensitive than behavioural, biochemical, or neuropathological measurements. Further research using direct comparison with other methods is needed to determine the conditions under which this is so and the significance of this in human risk assessment.

5. MORPHOLOGICAL METHODS

5.1 Introduction

5.1.1 Role of morphology

Just as neurobehavioural methods find their special use in the description and analysis of neurotoxic diseases for which there are no pathological correlates, the morphologist's special contribution is to describe neurotoxic conditions associated with structural alterations of nervous tissue (Table 2). Commonly, as in most chronic neurotoxic diseases, pathological alterations in the nervous system lead to changes in behaviour and function. These changes may provide important clues as to the site and even the nature of the underlying structural damage. Conversely, analysis of the location and type of pathological change often allows the morphologist to predict the type of accompanying dysfunction, the likely duration of the abnormality, and the degree of reversibility. This type of structural-functional correlation, so widely used in the evaluation of human neurological disorders, is especially helpful for assessing the severity of neurotoxic disease in experimental animals and, thereby, the implications for human exposure.

A properly conducted morphological examination of experimental animals establishes or rules out the existence of structural damage, identifies the most vulnerable sites within the nervous system and traces the temporal evolution of pathological changes. Armed with this information, the morphologist often is able to advise the electrophysiologist and biochemist where to focus their attention for the early detection and detailed analysis of the underlying neurocellular dysfunction.

5.1.2 Basis for morphological assessment

An understanding of the organization, structure, and function of the normal nervous system is the point of departure for any assessment of pathological changes induced by exposure to chemical substances. This requires not only a working knowledge of neuroanatomy (Williams & Warwick, 1975; Pansky & Allen, 1980), but also an understanding of structural variations that may occur in relation to factors such as the species under study and the age of the animal. In addition, since the morphologist usually studies dead tissue, an understanding of possible post-mortem changes is required.

Table 2. Morphological assessment in neurotoxic injuries

Type of neurotoxic injury	Chemical	Pathological change
Neurons		
excitable (neuronal) membrane	pyrethroid	none expected
neurotransmitter systems	anticholinesterase	none or terminal and muscle swelling
anabolic disturbance	doxorubicin	chromatolysis, or somal degeneration and neuronophagia, Wallerian degeneration, muscle atrophy (PNS), or transynaptic neuronal degeneration (CNS)
catabolic disturbance	swainsonine	increase of axonal and/or somal lysosomes
axonal transport	acrylamide	accumulation of cytoskeletal elements and/or organelles, Wallerian degeneration
dedrite	lathyrus toxin	swelling, variable involvement of soma
Special sense organs		
retina	methanol	oedema
inner ear	arsenical	degeneration of stria vascularis
Glial and myelinating cells		
astrocyte	6-aminonicotinamide	swelling and degeneration
oligodendrocyte	isoniazid	degeneration and myelin vacuolation
central myelin	triethyltin	myelin vacuolation and loss
Schwann cell	diptheria toxin	degeneration and local demyelination
peripheral myelin	hexachlorophene	myelin vacuolation and loss
Blood vessels		
	cadmium	haemorrhage and associated neurocellular degeneration

5.2 The Nervous System and Toxic Injuries

5.2.1 The nervous system

The nervous system may be separated anatomically into central and peripheral divisions. The peripheral nervous system (PNS) is composed of nerve cells (neurons) and their processes (axons) which conduct information between muscles, glands, sense organs, and the spinal cord or brain. The PNS includes afferent (sensory) and efferent (motor) fibres, and both types are represented in the somatic and visceral (autonomic) components of the nervous system. Somatic afferent fibres carry information from special organs and sensory receptors in skin and muscles, while visceral afferents convey impulses from the gut, glands, and various organs. On the motor side, somatic efferents innervate striated muscle, while visceral efferents supply smooth muscles of blood vessels, glands, and gut. In toxic states involving the PNS, degeneration of somatic sensory-motor fibres leads to peripheral neuropathies associated with sensory loss (e.g., decreased sensitivity to vibration, touch, and position sense) and motor weakness in distal extremities, while dysfunction or breakdown of autonomic fibres may lead to abnormal sweating, cardiovascular changes, or gastrointestinal, urinary-tract, genital, and other types of dysfunction (Schaumburg et al., 1983; Dyck et al., 1984).

Manifestations of central nervous system (CNS) disorders depend largely on the site and nature of the induced functional or structural change (Collins, 1982). The CNS consists of the parts of the nervous system contained within the skull and vertebral column. The spinal cord receives information from PNS afferents supplying skin, muscles, and glands, transmits signals for motor function by way of efferent fibres, and communicates via specific pathways with coordination centres within the brain. The brain is immensely complex and responsible for initiating, receiving, and integrating signals needed to maintain internal homeostasis, cognition, awareness, memory, language, personality, sexual behaviour, sleep and wakefulness, locomotion, sensation, vision, audition, balance, and many other body functions. Most of the available information on the structural-functional correlates of brain come from the study of higher mammals, including man (Truex & Carpenter, 1983). The brainstem, consisting of the midbrain, pons, and medulla oblongata, receives and processes information from skin, muscles, and special sense organs (e.g., inner ear) and, in turn, controls these muscles, as well as certain autonomic functions. The cerebellum and basal ganglia are required for the modulation and coordination of muscle movement. The diencephalon, including the thalamus and hypothalamus, is a relay zone for transmitting information about sensation and movement, and also contains important control mechanisms to maintain the internal homeostasis of the body. The hypothalamus functions as the primary control centre for the visceral system and serves to integrate the activity of the endocrine and other systems. The cerebral hemispheres, capped by the cerebral cortex, are concerned with perceptual, cognitive, motor, sensory, visual, and other functions. The optic nerves and their radiations conduct visual information from the retina, through the thalamus to the occipital cortex.

5.2.2 Cellular structure of the nervous system

Neurons and glial cells are the fundamental cellular elements of the nervous system, and these are associated with blood vessels and other specialized epithelial and connective tissue cells (Williams & Warwick, 1975). Neurons are equipped with multiple short processes (dendrites) that receive information from other nerve cells, and a single long axon that conducts electrical signals to other neurons and muscles, and to or from the skin, muscles, and glands (Fig. 1). The axon terminates at a synapse where chemically-encoded information is conveyed to neurons or muscle.

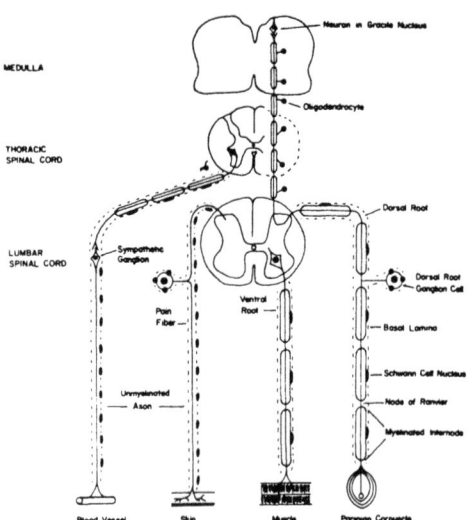

Fig. 1. The principal components of the peripheral nervous system (Schaumburg et al., 1983).

Glial cells in the CNS include astrocytes, oligodendrocytes, and microglia (Fig. 2). Astrocytes are divisible into protoplasmic and fibrous forms, are closely associated with neurons and blood vessels, and may play a nutritive role in maintaining neurons and other cells. Oligodendrocytes are responsible for elaborating short lengths of myelin around multiple axons, and microglia have a phagocytic function. In the PNS, Schwann cells envelop multiple small axons (unmyelinated fibres) or associate with and elaborate lengths of myelin (internodes) around single axons. Myelinated and unmyelinated fibres are separated from each other by endoneurial connective tissue composed of fibroblasts and collagen, and these elements are bound together in fasciles surrounded by a fibrocellular sleeve, the perineurium. Bundles of fascicles held together by epineurial connective tissue form a peripheral nerve.

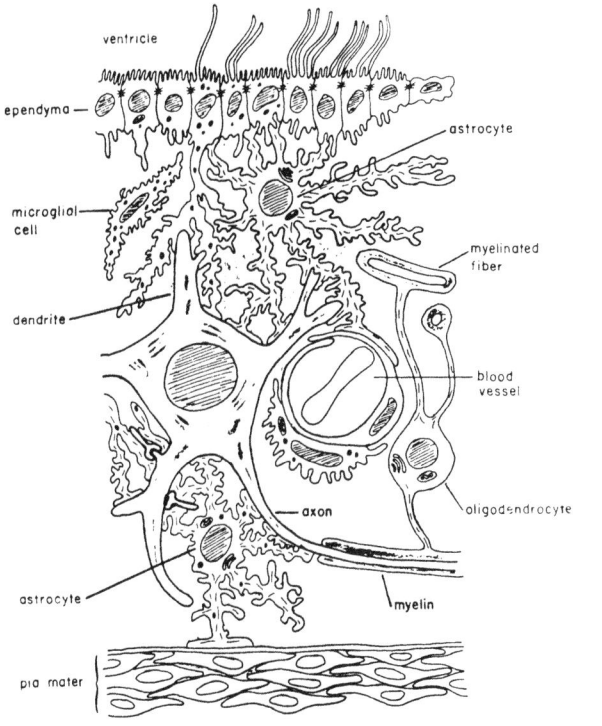

Fig. 2. Types of non-neuronal cells in the central nervous system (Williams & Warwick, 1975).

5.2.3 Neurocellular reaction to injury

5.2.3.1 Biological principles

Neurons are highly atypical cells because their cytoplasmic processes often occupy a much greater volume than their cell somata. This unusual cellular architecture provides an enormous surface area for chemical attack and places a great demand on the soma, since it alone has the metabolic machinery required to maintain the cellular processes. Specialized transport systems have evolved to convey information to the cell body, the axon, and its terminal regions (Ochs, 1982). The functional problem can be illustrated by considering a peripheral motor neuron, located in the lumbar spinal cord and innervating muscle in the foot, which must maintain the structure and function of an axon that is about a metre in length. Failure to maintain the entire length of this enormous column of cytoplasm, by interruption of axonal transport or by some other mechanism, may account for the vulnerability of distal axons in many types of neurotoxic disease. Other types of neurotoxins (e.g., doxorubicin) may interfere with the metabolic machinery of the soma, thereby resulting in degeneration of the entire neuron. Comparable explanations can be offered to explain the vulnerability to chemical attack of myelinating cells, their cytoplasmic processes, and myelin sheath (Spencer & Schaumburg, 1980).

There are two considerations when contemplating toxic damage to an organ or tissue. First, there are the changes that can be related to the action of the chemical agent; second, there is the reaction of the tissue to these changes. When toxic damage to neurons and myelinating cells is considered, it is often difficult to separate the two phases of the pathological process being studied. The situation is further complicated as the type of change observed is often dependent on dose, and may also vary with other factors, such as the species. In general, however, chemical attack leads to two types of primary change in neural cells:

(a) the accumulation, proliferation, or rearrangement of structural elements (e.g., intermediate filaments, microtubules) or organelles (e.g., mitochondria, lysosomes); and/or

(b) the breakdown (degeneration) of cells, in whole or in part.

The latter is usually followed by regenerative processes, and these may occur during the period of intoxication. Changes in the cellular elements of intraneural blood vessels may occur, and secondary changes may develop in other organ systems, notably voluntary muscle (Walton, 1974).

Neural cells appear to have a limited repertoire of pathological responses, and the consequences of many types of toxic damage can be predicted from an understanding of the biology and function of the cells that are involved. As in any organ system, changes in one cell type – the primary target – usually lead to secondary and tertiary responses in related cells, so that the net effect is a predictable cascade of pathological responses. For the nervous system, however, the neuropathological changes often have to be considered with regard to the fact that, while cellular responses to toxic injury may occur locally, they may also occur at distant sites. Changes may also develop in different locations as a function of time, dose, and/or duration of intoxication.

5.2.3.2 Neurons

Loss of the cell body of neurons (neuronopathy) is an irreversible event seen in many types of intoxication. Similar tissue reactions occur in the CNS and PNS. Fig. 3 illustrates the changes occurring with loss of primary sensory neurons in dorsal root ganglia. Glial cells and macrophages proliferate around the dying cell (neuronophagia) and axon processes under Wallerian degeneration. This involves breakdown of the entire length of the axon, dissolution and removal of the myelin sheath, and the proliferation of phagocytic and glial cells. Degenerated myelin is removed more slowly in the CNS than in the PNS and astrocytes increase the number and size of their fiberous processes to occupy the space left by the degenerating nerve fibre. Axon degeneration also produces significant secondary changes in the denervated cells, such as muscle (neurogenic atrophy) or other neurons (transynaptic and retrograde transynaptic degeneration) (Blackwood et al., 1971).

Neurons survive and recover from certain types of toxic assault, notably those that cause structural damage to their processes. Abnormalities of axons may be expressed in the form of generalized atrophy or localized swellings containing excessive numbers of structural elements or organelles, with associated secondary changes in the myelin sheath in the form of corrugation and displacement (secondary demyelination), respectively. Disruption of axonal integrity leads to axon atrophy and/or degeneration (axonopathy) below the site of injury (Fig. 4), with secondary changes in target cells, such as muscle (neurogenic atrophy) or neuron (transynaptic degeneration). Oligodendrocytes and Schwann cells lose their ability to maintain myelin and then undergo cell division,

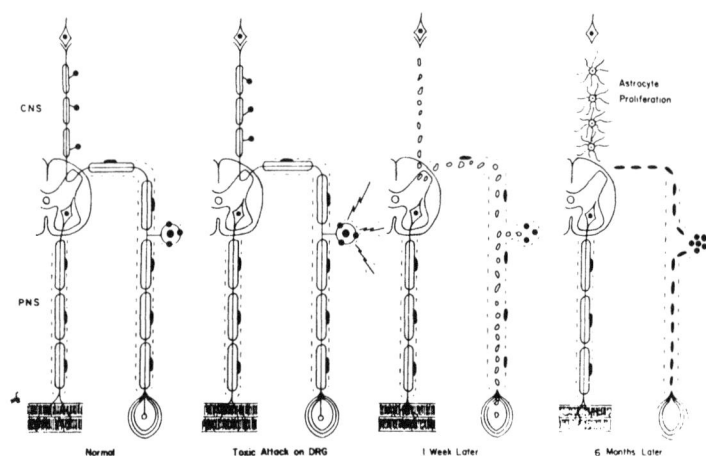

Fig. 3. The cardinal features of toxic sensory neuropathy. The "lightening bolts" illustrate that the toxin is directed at neurons in the dorsal root ganlion. Degeneration is accompanied by fragmentation and phagocytosis of peripheral-central processes. Schwann cells remain; there is no axonal regeneration.

while phagocytic cells remove the myelin debris. The cell bodies of affected neurons may also undergo responses secondary to axonal lesions, including cell necrosis or, more commonly, rearrangement of cellular components (chromatolysis) as a prelude to axon regeneration. Regrowth of the axon commences promptly at the position of axon interruption and, in the PNS, the elongating neuronal process reassociates with Schwann cells, which elaborate a new myelin sheath and conduct the regenerating axon to its target organ (muscle or sense organ) (Schaumburg et al., 1983). In the CNS, astrocytes respond to injury by increasing the number and size of their fibrous processes, and these appear to inhibit regeneration of all but the smallest (e.g., monoaminergic) axons. Prominent axon swellings develop at the viable end of larger fibres, a process known as axonal dystrophy.

5.2.3.3 Myelinating cells

Some chemical compounds induce primary morphological changes in myelinating cells or their myelin sheaths. It is usual to separate agents that induce changes in the cell body of Schwann cells or oligodendrocytes from those that cause

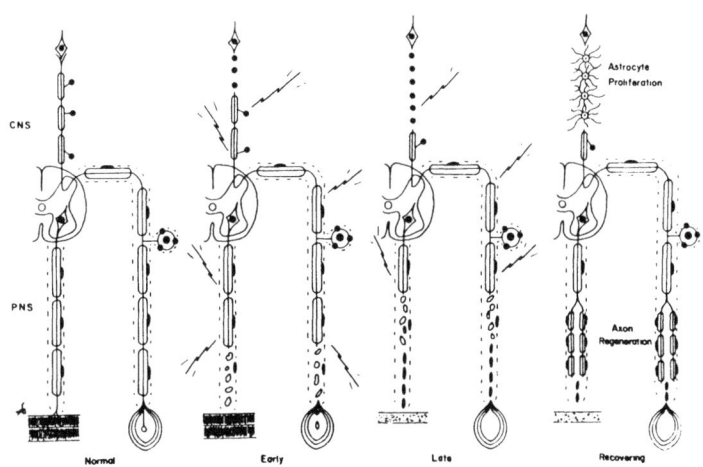

Fig. 4. The pathological features of toxic distal axonopathy. The "lightening bolts" indicate that the toxin is acting at multiple sites along sensory and motor axons of the central and peripheral nervous system. By the late stage, axon degeneration has moved proximally (dying-back). Central nervous system recovery is impeded by astroglial proliferation.

abnormalities selectively in the myelin sheath, though this distinction may be misleading as many compounds can produce both types of change, depending on dose and length of exposure. The net result of either type of CNS or PNS insult is primary demyelination (myelinopathy) (Fig. 5). Loss of oligodendrocyte somata is associated with the arrival of phagocytic cells which remove myelin and become filled with droplets of neutral fat. Astrocytes are commonly affected by chemical agents that perturb oligodendrocytes but, if they survive, astrocytes may also take up small amounts of myelin debris, divide, hypertrophy and, if remyelination does not occur, surround the demyelinated axons. More usually, however, new oligodendrocytes are recruited, their processes contact the demyelinated axon and these elaborate new but foreshortened internodal lengths of myelin (remyelination). Loss of Schwann cells also results in primary demyelination, cell multiplication, and remyelination. Another common type of myelinopathy involves the processes of CNS and PNS myelinating cells: these disorders are usually visualized by the accumulation of oedema fluid within the myelin sheath or its associated cellular processes (Spencer & Schaumburg, 1980). Vacuolation of the myelin sheath is usually a reversible process, though severe

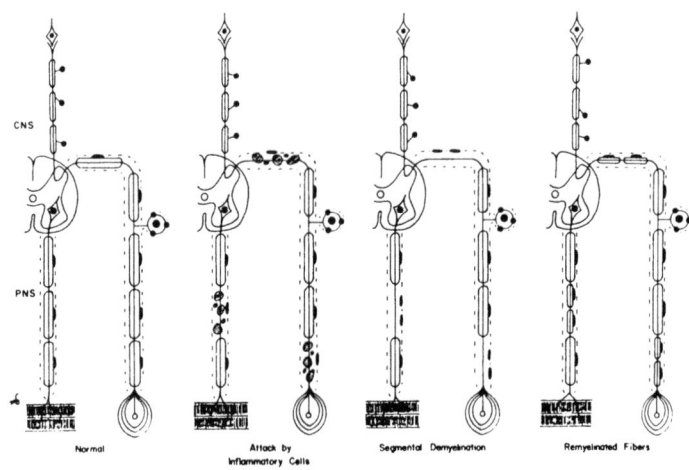

Fig. 5. The pathological features of an inflammatory peripheral nervous system myelinopathy. Axons and central nervous system myelin are spared. Following the attack, remaining Schwann cells divide and denuded axon segments are remyelinated with shortened internodes.

intramyelinic swelling may constrict the axon and induce Wallerian degeneration.

5.3 Experimental Design and Execution

5.3.1 General principles and procedure

Morphological examination is primarily concerned with studying structural changes in the nervous system that might explain behavioural disturbances. These changes are most commonly found when there is repeated dosing, but permanent neurological damage may also occur after single doses of some compounds. On occasion, such changes appear to be minor but, if restricted to a few neurons of a nucleus of considerable importance, may result in profound functional effects. This is particularly true of the developing nervous system where, because of stepwise, interdependent development, damage induced by a chemical agent at one stage may have a "domino effect" on later stages of development. Damage to CNS structures, especially when loss of nerve cells is involved, is more likely to be associated with permanent behavioural changes than disorders predominantly affecting the peripheral nervous system, where satisfactory regeneration is more often the rule. Rapidly reversible effects on behaviour are occasionally, but not often, associated with detectable structural damage to the nervous system.

5.3.2 Gross morphology

While most neurotoxic damage is most evident at the microscopic level, it is important to pay attention to the weight of the brain as well as to macroscopic manifestations such as discolouration (for example, due to bilirubin), discrete or massive haemorrhage, or other localized lesions (for example, transverse myelitis).

The new methods of nuclear magnetic resonance (NMR) can supply data concerning structural changes, for example, demyelination, both in vivo and post-mortem.

5.3.3 The role of histology

There is no substitute for a thorough light-microscope examination of the nervous system and other organs for the initial assessment of animals suspected of having neurotoxic injury. The same careful attention to anatomical detail should be given in the examination of experimental animal tissues as would be given by a pathologist studying autopsy tissue from a patient who has suffered from a new type of neurological disease. The results of this type of analysis will provide direction for additional studies that focus on more specific questions such as the type and extent of structural damage, the location where changes first occurred, the time-to-onset of structural damage, the reversibility of these changes, the lowest dose that caused pathological changes, and the highest no-observed-adverse-effect dose.

5.3.3.1 Biological principles dictating tissue response

The study design must take into account several important principles of underlying cellular reponses to injury. These principles will influence when and where tissue should be sampled for morphological study.

Often, there is a delay of days or weeks between dosing and the first appearance of structural changes in animals treated with neurotoxic agents. The extent of the delay depends largely on the chemical used, the dose, and the species studied. Once the pathological process has been initiated, a chain of degenerative and regenerative events may be set in motion, and these may or may not cease to evolve after dosing has stopped. Most neurotoxic substances that damage neurocellular elements produce a largely symmetrical pattern of structural change, whether in the CNS or PNS. Some neurons or nerve fibres may be more vulnerable than others to chemical attack, so that at any point in the pathological process, the observer may be presented with many or all of the stages in the reaction of individual cellular elements. The active pathological process may also move in space with time, as in dying-back axonpathies in which degeneration proceeds retrogradely along affected nerve and fibre tracts (Cavanagh, 1964). Careless sampling of animals with these or other types of neurotoxic diseases may reveal little or no pathological changes. By contrast, the careful and thorough investigator will be able to distinguish between early and later changes, and thereby develop a hypothesis of the spatial-temporal sequence of the pathological process. This can be tested in subsequent studies in which animals are examined at different stages in the development of the disease. Investigations of this type will also provide information on the relationship between the dose and duration of treatment required to induce neurotoxic injury. No-observed-adverse-effect levels can be established by determining doses that do not produce any characteristic changes after a specific period of chemical treatment. Quantitative estimation of structural abnormalities in treated versus control animals becomes increasingly important as the no-observed-adverse-effect dose is approached.

5.3.4   Use of controls

Parallel study of age-matched control animals is mandatory, whenever treated animals are subjected to neuropathological examination. Control groups should include untreated animals, vehicle-treated animals, and positive controls. The may receive a neurotoxic dose of the agent under study or of another compound with well-characterized neurotoxic properties that elicits a comparable type of neurotoxic damage. Demonstrating the development of an appropriate neurotoxic response in the positive control strengthens the validity of data obtained from animals treated with the agent under study, especially if these prove to lack pathological changes. The use of positive controls is imperative for the inexperienced investigator who needs to gain confidence from the self-demonstration that a known neurotoxic agent produces the expected changes. Inclusion of these results in a published report will also reassure the audience that the investigator has reproduced the expected pattern of structural damage associated with a known neurotoxic chemical.

There are important advantages in studying the structure of nervous tissue without knowledge of the treatment group. The investigator is forced to be more critical in seeking and describing abnormal findings, and the final assessment is a more objective statement of the similarities and differences between treatment and control groups.

5.3.5 Pattern of response

It is not the purpose of this publication to provide a detailed analysis of the various problems of selective neuronal damage encountered under neurotoxic conditions. However, it is emphasised that occasionally the localization is very precise, limited to one or two nuclei in the brain stem, or to distal regions of long fibre tracts and peripheral nerves. Selective pathological changes are given in Table 3 for reference in interpreting new situations.

5.3.6 Data acquired

At the end of the survey, clear answers must be found to the following questions about the CNS:

1. Are there changes in nerve cells in the area of the cerebral cortex, basal ganglia, hypothalamus, limbic system, diencephalon, brain stem, cerebellum, or spinal cord?

2. Are there any changes in shape or number of astroglia and/or microglial cells?

3. Is there any loss or other change in oligodendroglia?

4. Are there any changes in the myelinated areas of the brain or spinal cord, such as myelin fragmentation or myelin vacuolation? Is this associated with axonal swellings and/or degeneration?

5. If 4 is positive, are there glial responses?

6. Are there focal, vascular, and necrotic changes? If so, where?

7. Are tumours present?

8. Are there any changes in special sense organs to account for functional changes?

For the peripheral nerves, the following questions must be answered:

1. Are there any changes in peripheral nerves?

Table 3. Examples of toxic effects illustrating the specific patterns of damage that may be found

Pattern	Cause	Reference
Neuronal changes		
laminar cortical necrosis	anoxia	Brierly (1976)
hippocampal pyramidal cell damage	trimethylin	Brown et al. (1979)
selective granule cell loss from the cerebellum	methylmercury	Hunter & Russell (1954)
selective loss of inferior olivary cells	3-acetylpyridine	Desclin (1974)
selective degeneration of perikarya of sensory ganglion cells	doxorubicin	Cho et al. (1980)
selective degeneration of axons of sensory ganglion cells	methylmercury	Cavanagh & Chen (1971)
retrograde degeneration of long sensory and motor axons in CNS and PNS	organophosphorus, acrylamide, hexanedione	Cavanagh (1964); Spencer & Schaumburg (1977)
retrograde degenerations of axons of long spinal cord tracts	clioquinol	Krinke et al. (1979)
Myelin changes		
CNS myelin vacuolation	triethyltin	Aleu et al. (1963)
CNS and PNS myelin vacuolatin	hexachlorphene	Towfighi et al. (1975)
focal degeneration of PNS myelin without axon loss	diphtheria	Cavanagh & Jacobs (1954)
focal degeneration of PNS myelin with some axon loss	lead	Fullerton (1966)
Vascular and neurotic changes		
symmetrical lesions in brain-stem nuclei	misonidazole	Griffin et al. (1980)
non-symmetrical brain-stem and cortical lesions	lead	Wells et al. (1976)

2. If so, is it axon degeneration or primary demyelination, or both?

3. What is the distribution of degeneration? Is it distal, affecting only long and large-diameter fibres, or are shorter fibres such as cranial nerves also affected?

4. Are sensory, motor, or both types of fibres involved?

5. What is the state of nerve cell bodies (i.e., sensory ganglion cells, anterior horn cells)?

6. If the cells in 5 show changes, are those in the medulla and trigeminal ganglia (i.e., cranial nerves) similarly affected?

7. Are neurons normal, chromatolytic, or degenerated?

8. Are automatic ganglia or nerves similarly affected or not?

9. Are muscles affected by denervation and/or myopathic changes?

10. At dose levels below those that produce clinical signs, is there histochemical and/or morphometric evidence of metabolic neuronal changes that is brought out by using these more sensitive techniques?

5.4. Principles, Limitations, and Pitfalls of the Morphological Approach

5.4.1 Tissue state

Although under special circumstances the morphologist is able to study the reactions of living tissue to chemical exposure, either *in vivo* or in tissue culture (Yonesawa et al., 1980), the vast majority of pathological studies involve the assessment of dead tissue. The structural changes that occur in the nervous system as a function of time post-mortem can obscure the recognition of toxic injury and may confuse the inexperienced neuropathologist. Chemical, or rarely, physical (freezing) fixation methods are used to prevent the development of post-mortem changes.

5.4.2 Principles of fixation

The use of a reliable fixation method is mandatory for the morphological examination of nervous tissue (Thompson, 1963; Pease, 1964; Hayat, 1973; Gabe, 1976; Bancroft & Stevens,

1977; Glausert, 1980). The purpose of fixation is to preserve cellular architecture as closely as possible to that in the living state, to inhibit the loss of chemical components required for the maintenance of morphology, and to prepare the tissue to accept stains that enhance tissue density for clear resolution of cytological detail. The ideal method of fixation is one that instantaneously terminates life processes in the tissue of interest without distorting cytological detail. Rapid freezing of living tissue approaches this ideal. Excision and freezing of tissue is routinely employed for the assessment of human biopsy tissue and is particularly suitable for light-microscope histochemistry and immunocytochemistry. A few specialized laboratories use rapid freezing for the examination of tissue, or metal replicas thereof, by transmission electron microscopy.

Chemical methods are far more commonly used in neurotoxicology for the preparation of nervous tissue. Although the ideal chemical fixative should instantaneously kill living tissue without inducing structural changes, all known methods fall short of this ideal. Instead, the morphologist must strive to induce small, consistent and readily recognizable changes that will not compromise tissue examination and assessment. The most satisfactory and widely used chemical fixatives are dilute, aqueous solutions of aldehydes (formaldehyde and/or glutaraldehyde), which rapidly cross-link proteins and stabilize associated lipids, prevent post-mortem changes, and introduce rigidity into the tissue to facilitate handling. A secondary phase of fixation using a dilute aqueous solution of osmium tetroxide to fix lipids is routinely added after glutaraldehyde fixation for improved preservation of tissue. Occasionally, osmium tetroxide is used as the primary fixative. Structural artefacts induced by fixation are minimized if the fixative solutions are buffered to match tissue pH and osmolality. Temperature should also be controlled; low temperatures may affect the preservation of fine structural elements (e.g., microtubles).

Chemical fixatives must be delivered to the site of interest as rapidly as possible if post-mortem artefacts are to be minimized. Most effective is systemic perfusion (Pease, 1964; Hayat, 1973; Spencer et al., 1980; Spencer & Bischoff, 1982), in which the fixative is introduced via the ascending aorta of the deeply anaesthetized animal, and distributed throughout the vascular network under controlled pressure. Spaces normally occupied by blood and tissue fluid are rapidly replaced by the chosen fixative solution, and the animal expires painlessly within seconds. Perfusion of individual organs is an alternative, but more difficult and less satisfactory technique. An alternative method, suitable only for readily accessible parts of the nervous system (e.g., peripheral nerves), is to bathe the tissue in situ with a repeatedly replenished solution of fixative.

In practical terms, the requirements for tissue sampling, organ weighing, etc., have to be balanced against the need to get good fixation, and this frequently presents conflicts of interest between those involved in analysing the animal tissues. Short perfusion fixation (section 5.5.2), with paraformaldehyde and subsequent secondary fixation in formalin or formal-acetic acid in the case of paraffin sections and light microscopy, and glutaraldehyde and osmium tetroxide in the case of epoxy resin, semi-thin sections, may help to provide a compromise. When the protocol for killing requires only immersion fixation, then a few animals in each group must be kept for perfusion fixation, if adequate tissue examination is going to be achieved. A study using only immersion fixation is scarcely worth the labour and cost involved.

The selection of the chemical fixative and its method of delivery to the tissue site are chosen according to the type of information that is required. Systemic perfusion with the chosen fixative is always to be preferred. In general, formaldehyde is suitable for studies that require widespread tissue sampling, low resolution of cytological detail, or the use of special histochemical stains to assess the chemical content of abnormal cells and tissues. Conversely, in studies focusing on more selected areas of the nervous system or requiring resolution of fine structural detail, the use of glutaraldehyde and osmium tetroxide is mandatory. While the latter method was originally introduced for use in transmission electron microscopy, an increasing number of laboratories use the technique routinely to exploit the remarkable resolution afforded by the light microscope.

5.4.3 Principles of tissue sampling

Extensive sampling of tissue is essential for the initial assessment of a suspected neurotoxic injury. Organs, other than the nervous system, which should be examined, are listed in WHO (1978). Neural tissue should include: brain, including cerebellum, brain stem, pituitary gland, eye with occulomotor muscles and optic nerve attached, spinal cord, several sensory ganglia, sciatic nerve and its branches from its exit from the vertebral column to the level of the ankle, and selected muscles innervated by the sciatic nerve and its branches. Other regions less commonly sampled include: olfactory epithelium and tubercles, inner ear and labyrinths, plantar nerves and skin receptors, autonomic ganglia, and nerves and organs of innervation, such as the gut. The brain contains many sites known to be vulnerable to chemical agents and should be examined as thoroughly as possible. The use of an atlas such as that for the rat brain (Zeman & Innes, 1963) will be valuable. The brain stem should be sectioned just rostral to the cerebellum, the slice passing through the inferior colliculi. The cerebral hemispheres can then be sliced coronally (transversely). Olfactory lobes may be taken if questions of inhalation and olfaction are being studied. The cerebellum is removed by cutting through the peduncles that attach it to the brain stem. Sagittal sections are obtained by cutting through the midline, and parallel sections are also taken. Emphasis is usually placed on the retina and optic nerves, since these are often heavily involved in toxic diseases affecting neurons, axons, and myelin. Ototoxicity is also a common event, though the technical difficulties associated with the examination of the inner ear and labyrinths have prevented widespread study of this phenomenon. Olfactory lobes and associated epithelium are rarely examined, but should be taken if questions of inhalation and olfaction are being studied.

The spinal cord contains ascending and descending nerve fibre tracts that commonly undergo changes in myelinopathies and axonopathies (Table 3). Since the latter are tractable diseases with distal accentuation, it is critical to sample various levels from the medulla oblongata (where the gracile tract terminates) to the sacral region. By taking transverse sections of the spinal cord, it is possible to make a simultaneous evaluation of white matter (myelinated tracts and glial cells), gray matter (neurons, dendrites, proximal axons, glial cells), blood vessels, and associated tissues.

Dorsal root and cranial nerve ganglia contain primary sensory neurons that may display pathological changes in certain neuronopathies and axonopathies (Figs. 3, 4). Structural alterations in blood vessels and myelin may also occur under certain conditions. The sensory ganglia of the Vth cranial nerve, at least 4 sensory ganglia from the cervical bulb region (C5-T1 spinal levels), and 4 from the lumbosacral regions (L3-S2 spinal levels), should be sampled for examination in longitudinal section. Corresponding dorsal and ventral spinal roots, vulnerable in toxic demyelinating diseases, should also be studied.

Peripheral nerves commonly display changes in neurotoxic diseases affecting myelin, neurons, and axons (Table 3). As the last display distal, retrograde changes in dying-back axonopathies, a common response to chemical attack, it is critical to examine several levels of vulnerable nerves. Samples of the sciatic nerve and its branches are usually taken commencing adjacent to the vertebral column and terminating in the distal regions of the sural nerve, peroneal nerve, and/or the tibial nerve. The fine branches of the tibial nerve that leave the main trunk below the knee are especially vulnerable in toxic neuropathies, because they contain very large myelinated nerve fibres. Terminal regions of sensory and motor nerve fibres can be examined by searching for twigs supplying intrafusal (spindles) and extrafusal muscle fibres, respectively (Schaumburg et al., 1974). Routinely, anterior tibial muscles, and gastronemius with suralis muscles are examined. Muscle tissue is also valuable for assessing whether there is denervation atrophy, evidence of toxic myopathy, nerve sprouting, or other regenerative activity (Pearson & Mostofi, 1973).

Tissue sampling should not only be tailored to the goal of the study but also to the method of fixation. In general, blocks of tissue several millimeters thick may be taken if the tissue has been fixed with formaldehyde and is destined for paraffin embedding. For tissue fixed with glutaraldehyde, the relatively slow rate of penetration of osmium tetroxide necessitates the use of thin (1 μm) slices of tissue. It is often helpful to mark a small area of tissue (with Indian ink or a small cut) to maintain the orientation. Elongate structures, such as peripheral nerves and spinal cord, are most readily studied in transverse sections, though important information is acquired by complementary examination of longitudinal sections. Particularly informative for the identification of pathological changes in peripheral nerves is the technique of microdissection (teasing apart intrafascicular tissue), which yields long lengths of individual myelinated nerve fibres suitable for light microscope examination. Inspection of these preparations can demonstrate rapidly the presence of primary demyelination and remyelination and axonal degeneration and regeneration. The minor changes characteristic of early toxic neuropathies, readily missed in the examination of sections, can be easily detected by this method. Other parts of the nervous system are technically difficult to examine by microdissection because of the absence of a collagen network to support the individual nerve fibres.

While it is prudent to embed tissues in paraffin wax or epoxy resin promptly, regions that will not be examined immediately can be stored in a solution and at a temperature appropriate to the method of fixation. Loss of tissue quality will occur in proportion to the length of storage.

5.4.4 Preparation of tissue for examination

While gross tissue changes can be visualized with the naked eye or by examination with a stereoscopic binocular microscope, and surface detail can be resolved with the scanning electron microscopy, routine examination of cellular structure requires the use of tissue sections. This inevitably places severe limitations on the amount of tissue that is practical to study. Sections must be such that the energy beam (light, electrons, X-rays) of the chosen microscope can be transmitted through the tissue. Relatively thick sections containing several layers of cells can be visualized with the light microscope, but the ability to resolve cytological detail decreases as section thickness increases. The use of semi-thin sections allows the investigator to exploit the maximum available resolution of the light microscope. Much thinner sections are required for the assessment of tissue by transmission electron microscopy (Pease, 1964; Hayat, 1973).

Chemically-fixed tissue must be supported by a pliable material to facilitate the sectioning process and to prevent disintegration of the sectioned tissue. Paraffin wax or epoxy resin are routinely used: the former for routine work, the latter for more specialized studies. Since both types of embedding media are water insoluble and therefore immiscible with the fixative solutions, water is first removed by stepwise dehydration in ethanol or methanol immersing the tissue in an aromatic hydrocarbon (clearing solution) that is miscible both with ethanol and the embedding medium. Dehydration, clearing, and infiltration with an embedding medium are procedures requiring considerable care and time to avoid tissue drying and distortion. Automatic systems are available and, for paraffin embedding, these are routinely used in histological laboratories. Once the tissue is infiltrated and embedded, the medium must be allowed to harden by cooling (paraffin wax) or heating (epoxy resin).

Sections of tissue are prepared with the aid of knives mounted in microtomes. Steel knives are suitable to cut thick (4 - 15 μm) sections of paraffin embedded tissues, whereas knives prepared by scoring and breaking strips of special glass are needed to prepare sections (1 μm) of tissue embedded in the harder epoxy resin. The sections of tissue prepared with steel knives permits study of larger tissue areas than is possible with sections prepared from epoxy blocks, though the latter afford a higher resolution of cytological detail. With new developments in the preparation of glass knives and the design of microtomes, ever larger sections can be routinely prepared by the latter technique. Diamond knives mounted in ultramicrotomes are used to obtain the thin sections (50 nm) required for transmission electron microscopy.

Contrast of cytological detail in sectioned material can be enhanced by the use of special light-microscope methods (phase, Nomarski, fluoresence) or, more commonly, by the introduction of stains that render structures light-dense. A wealth of cytological stains is available for use with paraffin sections, whereas only a few general purpose stains are usually used to enhance structural detail for the light-microscope assessment of epoxy sections. Heavy metal stains that are electron dense are needed to visualize fine structure by transmission electron microscopy.

5.4.5 Recognition of artefact

Some degree of artefact is unavoidable, irrespective of the care taken in preparing tissue for morphological examination, and recognition and identification of the sources of artefact are of the utmost importance in the morphological assessment. Possible artefacts are legion and stem from various sources: e.g., poor tissue preservation from failure of fixative to penetrate tissue; shrinkage induced by inappropriate dehydration or drying; traumatic changes associated with excision of the tissue (bending, stretching) or rough handling during processing; wrinkling of sections and precipitation of stain (Spencer & Bischoff, 1982).

5.4.6 Recognition of normal structural variations

While the gross and fine structure of the nervous system of any species and age is remarkably constant from animal to animal, it is critical to recognize the irregular occurrence of normal variations in cellular structure that may lead the inexperienced observer to an inappropriate conclusion. These variations include ectopic structures (e.g., sensory neurons misplaced in the sciatic nerve), local oedematous or proliferative changes (e.g., at a site of unrecognized trauma or infection), and those that accompany advancing age (Johnson, 1981). The latter are especially important in long-term neurotoxicity studies, and there is no substitute for rigorous comparative study of control animals of the same age. Examples of normal age-related changes include neuronal pigmentation by lipofuscin, localized demyelination and remyelination, scattered neuronal loss, and axonal dystrophy and degeneration.

5.4.7 Qualitative versus quantitative approaches

While there can be no substitute for a thorough qualitative assessment of the morphological state of the nervous system, morphometric methods are required for a more precise description of these changes (Weibel, 1979; Bonashevskaya et al., 1983). This is especially important for the description of minor changes, or when the tissue reactions of different groups of animals are being compared. Randomization of samples is essential to minimize subjective influences, and a statistical approach is required both for the design of the morphometric study and the analysis of the data. Tissue sampling, group size, age, sex, body weight, and length are important considerations in this regard. This type of morphometric approach has been helpful in measuring tissue reactions to toxic chemicals in the form of: the numbers of fibres affected in specific pathways subject to degeneration, changes in cell populations in vulnerable parts of the brain, and the relationship between fibre diameter and internodal length of peripheral myelinated nerve fibres prepared by microdissection (Dyck et al., 1984).

5.5 Specific Procedures

5.5.1 Introduction

Strategic considerations in planning how to proceed must depend on the state of knowledge of the possible effects. When it is unknown whether damage occurs in nervous tissue, a wide-ranging examination of the nervous system with the light microscope is appropriate. Most structural changes induced by neurotoxic chemicals can be detected using the primary methods given below. More specialized, secondary methods can be applied subsequently for more detailed studies.

5.5.2 Primary methods

There are strong convictions among experienced experimental neuropathologists as to which fixation method should be chosen for the primary screening. Some believe the conventional approach using formaldehyde-based fixatives and paraffin embedding is most appropriate; others prefer the more contemporary method of examining epoxy sections of tissue fixed in glutaraldehyde and osmium tetroxide. Each method has significant advantages and disadvantages and both complement each other. Since it is impractical to use both methods for the same animal, a prudent investigator will include a sufficient number of animals to permit the parallel use of both procedures.

5.5.2.1 Formaldehyde/paraffin method

(a) Tissue fixation and excision

This technique is most suited for the study of large areas of tissue at low resolution and with special histochemical stains (section 5.5.3.3). Tissue can be removed from the carcass and fixed by immersion in formalin (10%) containing 2% acetic acid (added just before use) to improve penetration and hardening. Making up the solution in 80% alcohol rather than water to hasten penetration further has sometimes been recommended, but this is unnecessary and may make dissection more difficult.

Rapid and careful transfer of tissues from the carcass to the fixative solution will retard artefactual cell distortion. In a general post-mortem dissection, the brain, including the cerebellum and brainstem, are removed and transferred to fixative, prior to the removal of other tissues. Retrieval of the spinal cord from its spinal column is difficult and time consuming; it is recommended that the whole spinal column with cord be excised quickly, trimmed of as much muscle as possible, and immersed in the fixative intact. Once this portion is fixed, the spinal cord and ganglia can be separated from the column with greater care. Alternatively, after approximately 24 h of fixation, the spinal column can be immersed in 5% formic acid decalcifying solution. The column can then be sliced with little difficulty.

To assist with the examination of peripheral nerves, tissue is placed on a stiff card before immersion to retain orientation. Optimally, the nerve to be excised should be exposed and, prior to removal from the carcass, bathed with fixative for approximately 5 min. This will begin to introduce rigidity into the tissue and retard decay artefact. A length of nerve can then be excised, quickly placed on a card and pinned at the tip of both cut ends to retain position after immersion. Care should be taken to avoid overstretching the nerve as it is pinned to the card. Samples of these tissues can then be sectioned in a transverse or longitudinal direction. Muscle can be treated in the same manner. Another technique is to take off the limb at the hip or shoulder joint, remove the skin and fix en bloc in formalacetic acid solution. The limb can then be decalcified in 5% formic acid solution for approximately two weeks as noted earlier for the spinal column. It can then either be embedded in paraffin wax as one large block or further dissected.

Tissue preservation is greatly improved by perfusing animals systemically for 10 min with phosphate-buffered paraformaldehyde (section 5.5.2.2), a method that simultaneously preserves all body organs. Tissue can then be sampled in a more leisurely manner without fear of introducing post-mortem changes (section 5.5.2.2).

(b) <u>Dehydration and embedding</u>

Relatively large tissue samples can be embedded in paraffin wax, and this is particularly suitable for localizing and identifying lesions in the brain. Automated processing for paraffin embedding has greatly diminished the time requirements for preparing tissue samples. Most automated systems will conform to a variety of preparation schedules and process great numbers of tissue samples at one time. There are systems that operate under combined heat and vacuum, the great advantage being rapid processing. This combination is deleterious and may cause unnecessary shrinkage and brittleness, which will distort cell structure and hinder interpretation. Paraffin sections routinely cut 4 - 6 μm thick, are suitable for certain histochemical techniques and can easily be treated with special stain to enhance particular cellular components.

(c) Section staining

Four staining methods are routinely used to enhance cellular detail in paraffin sections.

Hematoxylin and eosin

Routinely used on paraffin sections, this method stains nuclei blue to purple, cytoplasm and Nissl substance (and mast cell granules) blue, and myelin sheaths pink. Nuclear density can be readily assessed, as well as an increase or decrease in the size of nuclei and the number of cells. Neuronal damage is readily detectable. Nuclei and cytoplasm of other cell types, such as microglia and vascular endothelial cells, are also well defined, though cresyl violet may be preferred.

Cresyl fast violet

This method enhances identification of cell-population changes and is more aesthetically pleasing than other basic aniline dyes, such as thionine or gallocyanine-chrome alum. DNA stains pale blue and RNA purple-blue. Hypertrophy of astroglial cytoplasm and changes in neuronal nuclei and cytoplasm are readily observed. Chromatolysis, poorly demonstrated in hematoxylin- and eosin-stained sections, is more apparent when stained with cresyl violet, as are most cells in peripheral nerves.

Glees and Marsland's stain

This method is easy to carry-out and selectively stains neurofibrillary components in axons (Marsland et al., 1954). Longitudinal sections demonstrate the state of terminal innervation in motor and sensory fibres. Empty endplates are often recognized by the observation of remaining clumps of nuclei on the muscle surface.

Sudan Black B

This method is useful to reveal nerve terminals in muscles (Cavanagh et al., 1964).

5.5.2.2 Glutaraldehyde/epoxy method

(a) Tissue fixation and excision

This technique is best suited for the resolution of early pathological changes with the light microscope and is required for transmission electron microscopy (section 5.5.3.5). Whole body perfusion with buffered fixators (paraformaldehyde) followed by glutaraldehyde) delivered under pressure (100 - 150 mm Hg) is the only satisfactory method to prepare brain and spinal cord sections, and this method has the advantage of optimally fixing all other organs simultaneously. For this purpose, the animal is deeply anaesthetized with a solution (e.g., sodium pentobarbital) containing a small percentage of heparin to facilitate circulation. Subsequent procedures should be performed rapidly and smoothly to prevent the development of anoxic damage and to ensure global fixation. The animal is secured on its back and the rib cage cut bilaterally and reflected backwards to expose the heart. After slitting the pericardium, the right atrium is opened to drain circulating blood. The ventricular apex is then excised to provide access to the aorta, and a cannula spurting a column of fixative is inserted through the ventricular opening to the apex of the aorta and clamped in place. The circulatory system is cleared by a brief, initial perfusion with paraformaldehyde or saline, and followed by more prolonged (e.g., 10 - 15 min) perfusion with glutaraldehyde.

Rigid tissues from a fixed carcass are less susceptible to handling artefact. The nervous system can be sampled in any order. In some laboratories, the entire nervous system, including brain with optic tract and nerves, spinal cord, spinal roots, ganglia, and peripheral nerves are exposed in the carcass, then carefully detached intact and removed. When this is accomplished, there is no need initially to mark tissues for orientation. It is imperative to avoid tissue drying during dissection and excision. Exposed tissues should be bathed with fixative and tissues should be manipulated as little as possible with forceps.

(b) Dehydration and embedding

After glutaraldehyde fixation, tissue samples are postfixed for 2 - 3 h by immersion in buffered 1 - 2% osmium tetroxide in the cold. The samples are then dehydrated stepwise in ascending concentrations of ethanol, immersed in acetone or toluene, infiltrated with a solution of epoxy resin and finally, embedded and polymerized in epoxy resin. For light-microscope examination, 1 μm sections are cut with specially prepared glass knives mounted in an ultramicrotome (an instrument designed specifically for the purpose of obtaining the thin sections suitable for electron microscope examination). New techniques and equipment have recently become available which allow larger tissue samples to be prepared for sectioning in epoxy resin. Sections one micrometer thick can be examined by phase-contrast optics or by bright field after a brief staining with 1% toluidine blue.

(c) Section staining

Thick (1 μm) sections of tissue fixed in glutaraldehyde and osmium tetroxide and stained with borate-buffered 1% toluidine blue allow resolution of structures as small as a single mitochondrion. Brain and spinal cord neurons display clearly defined nuclei, nucleoli, issl substance, and lipofuscin. Dendrites stand out against a more darkly-stained neuropil. Small, densely staining oligodendrocytes are readily distinguished from large, pale astrocytes. Myelinated nerve fibres contain a pale axon and darkly-stained myelin. In cross-sections of peripheral nerves, large and small diameter myelinated fibres, as well as the smallest unmyelinated axons, can be seen. Motor and sensory nerve terminals are detectable in muscle.

5.5.3 Special methods

5.5.3.1 Peripheral nerve microdissection

Isolated fibre preparations provide information that may be missed in cross-sections, and it is recommended that this procedure be included in any study concerned with toxic neuropathy. Several fixation methods are available to prepare peripheral nerves for microdissection. Perfused tissue is ideal, though satisfactory preparations can be obtained by bathing the tissue with fixative prior to excision. Post-excision immersion in fixative can also be used, though the act of transecting the nerve introduces major fibre artefacts that are not restricted to the cut ends and are readily mistaken for pathological changes.

Optimal preparations suitable for high-resolution light microscopy require the use of glutaraldehyde, post-fixation with osmium tetroxide, stepwise dehydration, and infiltration with a low-viscosity epoxy resin. This is an ideal medium to tease apart nerve fibres and is suitable for the storage of tissue at low temperature. Mounted fibres can be polymerized by heat to affix them to a glass slide and prevent squashing by a coverslip (Spencer & Thomas, 1970). Bright-field examination will reveal changes in overall structure, and Nomarski differential interference microscopy can be used to study the axon.

Older techniques yield poorer preservation, low resolution of detail, and isolated fibres are susceptible to squashing, an important consideration if morphometric study is planned. One method involves formalin fixation, post-fixation in osmium tetroxide, and infiltration with a dilute solution of glycerol, which is used to support the fibres during microdissection. Single fibres are mounted on the microscope slide, cleared with cresol, blotted dry, and mounted with pure glycerin (Thomas, 1970). Sudan Black B can also be used to stain tissue prior to microdissection. Nerves are microdissected with the aid of a pair of mounted needles and stereoscopic dissecting microscope. Epineurial connective tissue is removed and a small fascicle selected. After splitting the perineurium surrounding the fascicle, the sleeve is removed to expose the intrafascicular tissue containing the nerve fibres. The tissue is then repeatedly split into progressively smaller longitudinal bundles until individual fibres are obtained. These are picked up on the end of sharpened wooden applicator sticks and transferred to a clean glass slide and provided with a coverslip. Alternatively, a rapid "squash" preparation can be obtained by teasing a small bundle of fibres loosely apart to create a mesh formation on a microscope slide; a coverslip is then added for microscope examination.

5.5.3.2 Frozen sections

Frozen sections lend themselves well to enzyme histochemical, immunocytochemical, and silver-impregnation procedures, but for the purposes of a large-scale study, this method is impractical. Tissues fixed instantaneously by immersion in liquid nitrogen are particularly vulnerable to cell distortion and/or destruction caused by excessive temperature changes. Encasing tissue samples in gelatin or albumin is advisable, especially for brain tissues (Crane & Goldman, 1979). Ice-crystal formation is a disruptive artefact that produces a vacuolated appearance in frozen sections. To minimize crystal formation, it is important to freeze tissues as rapidly as possible and maintain critical temperatures throughout the cutting procedure to avoid thawing and refreezing. Typically, frozen sections are between 10 and 15 μm thick.

5.5.3.3 Histochemical methods

Using these procedures, it is possible to assess the activity of cell energy systems, the rate of use of substrates for processes of oxidative phosphorylation, and the functional state of intracellular organelles. The activities of succinate dehydrogenase and malate dehydrogenase, enzymes of the Krebs cycle, are well known, the former being closely linked with mitochondrial membranes. Enzymes of the hexose monophosphate shunt (glucose-6-phosphate dehyrogenase and gluconate-6-phosphate dehydrogenase) and those of the electron transport chain (NAD and NADP disphorase) should also be studied. The rate of exchange of nitrogenous bases can be examined by the determination of activity of dihydroorotate dehydrogenase for fatty acids; monoamine oxidase for biogenic amines; and acetylcholinesterase for acetylcholine.

Histochemical enzyme assays are performed on freshly frozen sections cut on a cryostat (Dubowitz & Brooks, 1973). Tissues are quick-frozen in liquid nitrogen. Control and experimental tissues should be mounted on one slide and reactions carried out using the methods outlined in Pearse (1968).

The following methods can be used to demonstrate the functional state of nerve cells (Pearse, 1968):

(a) RNA (Brachet's method with ribonuclease control);

(b) DNA (Feulgen's method with deoxyribonuclease control);

(c) Total nucleic acids (Einarsen's method);

(d) Total protein (sublimate with bromophenol blue);

(e) Sulfhydryl groups (Barnet and Zeligman's method);

(f) Glycogen and glycosaminoglycans (amylase control-PAS reaction); and

(g) Lipids (Sudan III, Sudan Black, Nile Blue methods).

To express histochemical reactions quantitatively, the following formula for Mean Histochemical Index (MHI) can be used:

$$MHI = \frac{3a + 2b + 1c + 0d}{N}$$

where 3, 2, 1, and 0 are the degrees of intensity of colour (from 3 to 0), and a, b, c, and d are the numbers of the cells with the given intensity of colour; the denominator N is the number of cells counted. The results allow statistical calculation of the assays and estimation of the reliability of the results.

5.5.3.4 Golgi method

This unique silver-impregnation method demonstrates the shape and surface characteristics of entire neurons, including cell bodies and their processes. Golgi preparations are particularly useful in the study of dendritic arborizations and synaptic associations (Santini, 1975). However, the technique is capricious in that only a few neurons are unpredictably demonstrated; many preparations must therefore be examined to gather a representative sample.

In the Rapid Golgi method, tissue is fixed with formaldehyde or glutaraldehyde and post-fixed with osmium tetroxide. The tissue is then impregnated with silver nitrate, dehydrated, and infiltrated with celloidin. Thick (120 µm) sections are prepared, mounted, and examined by bright-field microscopy.

5.5.3.5 Transmission electron microscopy

This technique is laborious and requires extensive training. However, it has resulted in extensive advances in the understanding of cellular processes in neurotoxicity. There is little need for such exacting methods to determine the presence of changes in cell structure, few experimental protocols require electron microscopy. The transmission electron microscope is properly used to confirm and study further the nature of lesions already shown and mapped by light microscopic methods. It is all too easy to seek, and find, changes to which no significance will ultimately be attached. Until the pattern of change induced by the chemical under study has been well identified by light microscopy, electron microscopy should not be considered. On rare occasions, such as in toxic disorders of unmyelinated axons, examination by transmission electron microscopy is necessary to localize cellular changes not revealed by the methods discussed previously. Thin (50 nm) plastic sections are prepared with the aid of a diamond knife mounted in an ultramicrotome and subsequently impregnated with heavy metals for electron-microscope examination (Pease, 1964; Hayat, 1973).

5.5.3.6 Other anatomical methods

There are numerous additional specialized anatomical methods that are waiting to be applied in the study of neurotoxicological issues. These include histological techniques to trace anatomical pathways (with horseradish peroxidase) and cellular activity. Examples of the latter are the use of autoradiography to localize the distribution of radiolabelled precursors such as thymidine and 2-dexoyglucose (Sokoloff et al., 1977). Other methods susceptible to light and electron microscope analysis include immunocytochemical studies of receptors, proteins, and other cell structures (Emson, 1983). Fluorescence microscopy, particularly for the localization and detection of regional concentrations of catecholamines using the formaldehyde vapour or glyoxylic acid technique of Falck et al. (1962), supplements quantitative biochemical methods in evaluating alterations in catecholamine levels. Fluorescence microscopy is also of value in antigen and antibody localization techniques. Certain light and electron microscope techniques may be combined, such as the examination of fine structure of single teased nerve fibres (Spencer & Lieberman, 1971; Ochoa, 1972) or of Golgi-stained preparations. Advanced methods in electron microscopy include scanning (for surface features), energy-dispersive X-ray analysis (for detection of elements of high relative atomic mass) and energy-loss (for detection of elements of low atomic mass). Freeze-fracturing tissue can reveal details of the internal surfaces of cellular membranes when replicas are examined by transmission electron microscopy (Hayat, 1973).

5.6 Conclusions

The information derived from morphological studies is highly relevant to the interpretation of biochemical, neurophysiological, and behavioural data. Structural changes have always been the firm foundation on which analysis of clinical neurological disease has been based. Both diagnosis and prognosis depend heavily on previous neuropathological experience for their accuracy. Moreover, treatment of neurological disease can only be satisfactorily planned by using the knowledge gained from experimental and morphological studies that have provided an understanding of the pattern by which neural cells are affected. Indeed, in the majority of human intoxications of the nervous system, knowledge of the structural changes is based almost exclusively on animal studies. There is no reason to believe that it will be less so in the future.

6. BIOCHEMICAL AND NEUROENDOCRINOLOGICAL METHODS

6.1 Introduction

Biochemical tools are valuable for the study of neurotoxicity. They have the potential for both identifying toxic compounds and delineating mechanisms of action of known toxic substances. However, the range of biochemical techniques is vast and careful decisions must be made in devising an effective research strategy. The most important decision is identification of the objective of the research, which may be conveniently categorized into three groups: determining mechanisms of action of neurotoxic substances, identifying exposed individuals, and screening for toxic conditions.

Devising an effective biochemical screen is the most challenging of the three objectives. It requires the selection of biochemical parameters that are general enough to indicate toxicity resulting from multiple sites of damage, but specific enough to prevent the accumulation of false positives. No single biochemical parameter is likely to suffice. An effective screen must include indices of each of the major functions of nervous tissue (e.g., cellular metabolism, neuronal propagation, and neurotransmission). It might include estimates of RNA and/or protein synthesis, lysosomal enzymes, membrane transport, channel and neurotransmitter receptors, or their turnover. The precise choice of biochemical indices must be limited by the expertise and equipment of individual laboratories, but every attempt must be made to consider a range of functional events rather than a single parameter.

Considerable discussion has centred on the use of _in vitro_ procedures for screening potential neurotoxic compounds. The advantages of an _in vitro_ approach are obvious. It is less expensive and less time-consuming than whole animal study and biochemical techniques can be employed under precise, standard conditions. _In vitro_ procedures must include both parent compounds and potential toxic metabolites. However, the exclusive use of _in vitro_ methods would fail to detect compounds in which the neurotoxicity results from alterations in non-neuronal systems.

Theoretically, the choice of biochemical tools for the identification of mechanisms of toxicity is the simplest of the three objectives. Biochemical tools are virtually limitless, but they can be chosen on the basis of known information about the toxicity of the compound. Scientists can then proceed systematically from one level of analysis to another. By synthesizing data from behavioural, neurophysiological, neuroendocrinological, neuropharmacological, and neuropathological studies, the biochemist can employ successively more selective tools to determine the initial biochemical lesion induced by the toxic compound.

The purpose of this section is to review the biochemical approaches that may be useful for identifying and further understanding the effects of toxic compounds on the nervous system.

6.2 Fractionation Methods

Neural tissue has several features not shared by other tissues. In particular, neural tissue exhibits considerable cellular, morphological, and chemical heterogeneity. It is often desirable to precede biochemical procedures with some attempt to decrease this complexity. One approach is to separate the tissue into discrete parts of brain prior to analyses. A second approach is to separate specific cell types. A third involves subcellular fractionation procedures. In many cases, it may be desirable to use a combination of these fractionation procedures.

6.2.1 Brain dissection

Brain tissue can be fractionated into any number of potential sections. However, the most often used scheme is based on that described by Glowinski & Iverson (1966). In this method the brain is divided into relatively discrete units of cerebellum, thalamus, hypothalamus, striatum, hippocampus, etc., by using visible anatomical landmarks. Such dissection procedures have been very useful in describing the neurochemistry of different brain areas and are essential in evaluating the effects of toxic compounds on molecules (such as neurotransmitters) that are not uniformally distributed in neural tissue. Because of the regional variability of brain chemistry, whole brain analyses are seldom useful for evaluating brain function. More importantly, the use of the whole brain for studies of toxic compounds may fail to detect functionally-relevant alterations in specific brain areas. For example, effects of lead on GABA levels have been reported for cerebellar tissue (Silbergeld et al., 1980) and acrylamide effects have been noted in striatal dopamine receptors (Bondy et al., 1981).

Differences in the response to toxic compounds would be anticipated from differences in neurochemistry in various regions of the brain. In addition, many toxic substances are not distributed uniformly across brain areas (e.g., chlordecone (Fujimori et al., 1982) and manganese (Bonilla et al., 1982). Although not predictive, examination of such regions can provide a biochemical clue regarding possible molecular sites of interaction of the toxic compounds.

In more precise dissection procedures, a small needle, of defined diameter, is used to obtain samples within anatomically defined areas (Palkovits, 1973; O'Callaghan et al., 1983). Such finite samples have been used in identifying several neurochemical events, e.g., neurotransmitter concentrations (Palkovits, 1973) and neurotransmitter-induced phosphorylation of specific phosphoproteins (Dolphin & Greengard, 1981), and they may be especially valuable in locating the site of neural responses to toxic compounds.

6.2.2 Isolation of specific cell types

Although neural tissue is recognized by a marked heterogeneity of cellular elements, based on function and embryonic origin, these cell types are conveniently categorized as neurons or glia. Each cell type makes a unique contribution to neural function and their sensitivity to toxic compounds may differ. Several methods have been described for the bulk separation of neuronal and glial cell populations from whole brain or specific brain regions (Rose & Sinha, 1970; Appel & Day, 1976; Magata & Tsukada, 1978). A dissociated cell suspension that avoids disruption of the cells is prepared by forcing the tissues through fine sieves. Proteolytic enzymes are used to facilitate the dissociation. The fraction enriched in neuronal perikarya is separated from the smaller glial cells (also containing some synaptosomes) by centrifugation. The cell separations are never complete and the procedures generally provide low yields. However, enrichment of the neurons and glia is usually sufficient for determining whether a toxic agent interferes primarily with neuronal or glial metabolism. Isolated cell populations have been used to study the lipid and protein composition of membranes and the several metabolic differences between neuron and glia. Such information may provide baseline data for future studies of neurotoxic chemicals. Disadvantages of this method include loss of cell processes from the perikarya, reduction of cell surface area, and damage to the cell membrane. These factors must be considered in any metabolic study.

To date, there have been few attempts to use such separation procedures in neurotoxicity and they are not recommended as an initial study. The method is laborious and time consuming and must be performed on fresh tissue. Only a limited number of samples can be simultaneously processed and it is never clear if the low yields result from random or specific loss of cell types.

6.2.3   Subcellular fractionation

The neuron can be divided into relatively discrete functional units. The cell body contains the metabolic machinery for the synthesis and packaging of macromolecules and for the general maintenance of cellular homeostatis. The long axonal process acts as a communication link, propagating electrical impulses from the cell body to the terminal and transporting vital nutrients and cellular components to more distal regions including the nerve terminal. Finally, the synapse functions to transfer chemically encoded information from one cell to another. Toxic substances may disrupt neuronal biochemistry at any one, or all, of these cellular sites.

The isolation of subcellular organelles and specific membrane fractions can be a first approximation in determining the subcellular sites of action of toxic agents. Differential centrifugation procedures provide a rapid means of obtaining fractions consisting predominantly of a single cellular component (Gray & Whittaker, 1962; Cotman & Barker, 1974; Rose and Sinha, 1970). Subcellular fractionation is never totally effective, but it can produce an enrichment of organelles and cellular subfractions. Some of the more commonly used biochemical markers that can help identify the degree of enrichment are listed in Table 4. These markers can be used as potential indices of toxicity. For example, the effects of triethyltin on myelination in the developing brain has been studied by examining the activity of the myelin marker, 2',3'cyclic nucleotide 3' phosphohydrolase (Konat & Clausen, 1977). Merkuryva & Tsapkova (1982) have used several marker enzymes in their study on the toxic effects of ethanol on the nervous system.

When subcellular fractionation is combined with regional analysis, the number of potential samples requiring examination can be overwhelming. Therefore, careful selection must be used in deciding which brain area and which subcellular fraction to investigate. This selection can be very difficult, especially when knowledge concerning a particular compound is limited. The recent introduction of immunochemical methods promises to facilitate this task, not by reducing the difficulty of the selection, but by increasing the number of chemicals that can be subjected for analysis.

Immunochemical methods have been used to identify molecules associated with various cell types, for localizing enzymes responsible for the synthesis of neurotransmitters. and for identifying proteins specific to the nervous system. While the procedures initially require the preparation of antisera to highly purified proteins, once the antisera are available, they can be sensitive tools for identifying

Table 4. Examples of biochemical markers of brain subcellular fractions and cell types

Fraction	Marker	Reference
nuclei	DNA	Steele & Busch (1963)
nuclear membrane	RNA polymerase	Roeder & Rutter (1969)
cytosol	lactate dehydrogenase	Kornberg (1955)
microsomes	NADPH: cytochrome c oxidoreductase (rotenone insensitive)	Miller & Dawson (1972)
Mitochondria		
inner membrane	D-3-hydroxybutyrate NAD^+ oxidoreductase	Fitzgerald et al. (1974)
outer membrane	monoamine oxidase	Schnaitman et al. (1967)
lysosomes	β-glucuronidase	Fishman & Bernfeld (1955)
	β-glucosidase	Robins et al. (1968)
	β-galactosidase	Robins et al. (1968)
	N-arylamidase	Boer (1974)
myelin	2',3'-cyclic nucleotide-3'-phosphohydrolase	Konat & Calusen (1977)
synaptosomes	Na^+K^+-activated oubain-sensitive ATPase	Verity (1972)
neuronal cells	guanyl cyclase tyrosine hydroxylase	Goridis et al. (1974) Kuczenski & Mandell (1972)
oligodendroglial cells	glyceride galactosyl transferase	Radin et al. (1972)

specific changes and for characterizing different cell populations. In addition, monoclonal antibodies can be used to determine the mechanism of action of toxins.

These procedures are especially valuable in studying neuronal peptides. These peptides (e.g., substance P, encephalins, hypothalamic releasing factors, somatostatin, etc.) play a significant role as neuromodulators (Snyder & Inms, 1979). Many are potent at low concentrations. Prior to the use of immunological procedures, peptide molecules could only be examined by using bioassay techniques and these were not always specific for particular molecular species. Radioimmunoassay techniques are more specific. Assay kits for various peptides are now available commercially, and their number is rapidly increasing.

Because the method is very recent, radioimmunoassay procedures are only beginning to be use in neurotoxicology. However, using such methods, Hong and his colleagues (Ali et al., 1982; Hong & Ali, 1982) have successfully identified several peptide responses following chlordecone treatment. The major limitation of the method for identifying toxic compounds is the small number of purified compounds, the small number of available RIA kits, and the expense of obtaining radioiodinated compounds. With increasing availability of RIA kits, the procedure could become a powerful screening tool.

6.3 DNA, RNA, and Protein Synthesis

Changes in the amount of DNA can be used to detect whether toxic agents affect cellular proliferation and cell death. Polyploidy is uncommon in the nervous system, thus the DNA content of brain regions can be taken as an index of cell number. This can be related to tissue weight and RNA or protein content to estimate cell size. For example, Krigman & Hogan (1974) reported that lead exposure during early development reduced brain weight and decreased total brain proteins, but the number of brain cells was unchanged. DNA measurements have been particularly useful in studying the toxic effects of drugs on retinal photoreceptors (Dewar et al., 1977). It is also well-known that the DNA content changes after nutritional restriction during development, or after exposure to various toxic chemicals that influence nutritional status.

Although the measurement of DNA content is relatively simple and in the nervous system can be an index of cell number, it is probably not a very sensitive or early indicator of neurotoxicity. For example, neuronal loss might be accompanied by glial proliferation and produce no change in total DNA. The earliest effects of a toxic substance on DNA will probably involve: (a) the disturbance of DNA-repair enzymes; (b) the intercalation of the substance into the DNA molecule; or (c) the direct binding of the substance to the nucleic acid moiety or its associated chromosomal proteins. Two to three percent of added mercuric chloride was reported to bind to the chromatin in cultured glial cells (Ramanujam et al., 1970). Since this mode of action will ultimately interfere with the functional integrity of the CNS, it offers great promise for the identification of toxic compounds.

The total amount of RNA or protein could also be examined after toxic insult. However, neither total RNA nor total protein is likely to provide a sensitive index of toxic damage. Only in the extreme stages of neurotoxicity will total or even regional levels of these macromolecules be likely to change. More sensitive indices of their metabolism rely on estimates of synthesis or degradation.

The rate of RNA or protein synthesis can be evaluated by using radiolabelled precursors and measuring their rate of incorporation into the macromolecule in vitro or in vivo. Although this technique is simple and sensitive, it assumes that the rate of incorporation of the precursor directly reflects the rate of macromolecular synthesis and this may not always be true (Dunn, 1977). Changes in labelling could also occur as a result of changes in cerebral blood flow, precursor transport, precursor pool size, energy charge, etc. Inhibition of amino acid transport across the blood-brain barrier has been reported for mercury (Partridge, 1976) and lead (Lorenzo & Gerwitz, 1977). Thus, it is also important to consider whether a toxic agent can cause changes in the amino acid or nucleic-acid-precursor pool sizes by using one of several methods available for compensating for precursor pool fluctuations (Munro et al., 1964; Dunlop et al., 1975; Dunn, 1975). Changes in brain-protein synthesis have been reported after exposure to methylmercury (Verity et al., 1977), and carbon disulfide (Savolaiene & Jarvisalo, 1977). However, in many cases, only the absolute levels of incorporation of radioactive amino acids into protein fractions were studied and it is difficult to understand the primary mechanisms of action.

Although these relatively crude methods are subject to several criticisms, all the variations that influence the incorporation of the radioactive precursor can ultimately influence cellular metabolism. These methods can, therefore, be useful for identifying metabolic disturbances. The relative amount of protein synthesis can also be estimated simply by measuring the polyribosome to free ribosome pool. This method is based on the assumption that during high rates of protein synthesis, the greatest proportion of the total ribosomes will be attached to an mRNA molecule. The relative polyribosome to monosome ratio has the advantage of allowing for normalization across animals and therefore reducing the interanimal variability that often plagues neurochemical assessments. Furthermore, the use of this method would detect toxic effects not only on protein synthesis but on the stability or synthesis of the ribosome itself.

The rate of RNA and protein synthesis in the brain is very high and nerve cell functioning is dependent on protein metabolism. The turnover rates of brain macromolecules may vary considerably, and it is always going to be difficult to interpret any data dealing with the turnover of total RNA or protein. However, with the availability of newer separation methods for proteins (detergent gel electrophoresis combined with chromatofocusing cellulose ion exchange chromatography, etc.), soluble and bound polypeptides can be separated to study the synthesis of individual proteins at the subcellular level, in specific cell types and in localized brain regions. Large classes of RNA can be analysed by hybridization procedures or specific mRNA molecules could be targeted for investigation by using specific cDNA probes.

6.4 Lipids, Glycolipids, and Glycoproteins

Complex lipids, glycolipids, and glycoproteins have several important functions in neural tissue (Zuber, 1978). They constitute structural elements of the plasma membrane, act as components of ion channels, comprise portions of neurotransmitter receptors, and are major constituents of myelin. Complex lipids (e.g., phospholipids, cerebrosides, sulfatides, and gangliosides) make up neuronal membranes. Phosphatides (phosphatidylethanolamine, phosphatidylcholine, phosphatidylinositol, phosphatidylserine) are the most important group of phospholipids. They consist of some of the most metabolically active of the phospholipids (Prokhorova, 1974) and participate in the movement of Na and K ions through the neural membrane. A closely related group of phospholipids, the plasmalogens, are concentrated in myelin and constitute 18 - 30% of total brain phospholipids.

Ganliosides are localized primarily in the plasma membrane (Karpova et al., 1978), but small amounts of monosialoganglioside are detectable in myelin. Receptors of neurotransmitters, such as serotonin, and other biologically-active compounds may contain ganglioside (Avrona, 1971), and evidence suggests that gangliosides may bind biologically-active compounds, as well as various neurotoxins, through their terminal N-acetylneuraminic acid moiety (Kryzhavosky, 1973). Glycosaminoglycans are also functional and structural elements of the neuronal membrane and have been reported to exhibit disturbed metabolism in various hereditary diseases of the mucopolysaccharidosis type (Constantopoulos et al., 1976; Vasan & Chase, 1976).

The most interesting of the functionally-active, minor components of neuronal membranes are sialic acids, and particularly N-acetylneuraminic acid. As sialo-glycoproteins and gangliosides, N-acetylneuraminic acid participates in carrying out specific neuronal functions such as the establishment of synaptic contact neurotransmission, and axonal propagation (Partingron & Daly, 1979). Gangliosides and sialo-glycoproteins bind Ca^{++} at their hydrophilic ends and thus, by influencing the concentration of this ion, affect depolarization and neurotransmitter release.

Myelin metabolism may be affected by a variety of toxic agents (Cammer, 1980). After administration of these compounds, there is often a delay before the appearance of neurotoxic signs and symptoms such as the ataxia indicative of peripheral demyelination. Central demyelination often occurs to a lesser extent. Compounds that cause disturbances in myelin metabolism may exert their effect directly on myelin-forming cells, or demyelination may be a secondary response to a disturbance of neuronal metabolism.

Several compounds have been reported to alter complex lipids or their metabolism. Neonatal exposure to lead has been reported to decrease the total brain content of phospholipids, galactolipids, plasmalogens, and cholesterol (Van Gelder, 1978). Hydrogen sulfide and sulfur dioxide decrease total brain lipids and/or phospholipids (Haider et al., 1980). Meta-Systox[R] (phosphorothioic acid O-[2-(ethylthio)ethyl] O,O-dimethyl ester mixture with S-[2-(ethylthio)ethyl] O,O-dimethyl phosphorothioate) (O,O-dimethyl-S-2 (ethylsulfinyl) ethylthiophosphate), an organophosphorus pesticide, has been reported to decrease brain levels of total lipids, phospholipids, cholesterol, esterfied fatty acids, and gangliosides (Islam et al., 1983). Merkuryva et al. (1978) found one of the early affects of carbon disulfide intoxication to be changes in the enzyme substrate system of N-acetylneuraminic acid,N-acetylneuraminate lyase. In the olfactory bulb of the rabbit, carbon disulfide led to an accumulation of N-acetyl-neuraminic acid because of a reduced degradation by β-acetyl-neuraminate lyase. In some cases, the carbon disulfide-induced disturbance of the metabolism of cerebral glycoconjugates could be correlated with the changing of physiological parameters (e.g., lowering of the amplitude of the cortical evoked potential (Bokina et al., 1976)). Long-term exposure to lead acetate in aging rats was reported to decrease N-acetyl-neuraminic acid content in cerebral tissue and also to decrease the activity of the degradative enzyme (Merkuryva & Bushinskaya 1982). Long-term exposure to ethanol led to an accumulation of N-acetylneuraminic acid in the subfornical region of the hypothalamus and in the midbrain reticular formation (Merkuryva et al., 1980).

A recently applied approach to the study of neurotoxicology involves the investigation of lipid peroxidation. Peroxidation involves the direct reaction of oxygen and lipids to form free radical intermediates and semistable peroxides. Lipid peroxidation is damaging because of the subsequent reactivity of these free radicals (Tappel, 1970). Biomembranes and subcellular organelles are the major cellular components damaged by lipid peroxidation. Increased lipid peroxidation has been reported after exposure to thallium, nickel, or cobalt (Hasan & Ali, 1981). Since the estimate of lipid perioxidation is a relatively simple technique, this method may prove to be an effective tool for screening for neurotoxic compounds.

6.5 Neurotransmitters

Chemical synaptic transmission involves a complex series of events (synthesis and storage of neurotransmitters, release of neurotransmitters, re-uptake or degradation of transmitters, interaction of transmitters with postsynaptic membrane), any or all of which could be disturbed by neurotoxins. In addition to the classical neurotransmitters (Table 5), a number of peptides have been discovered, which may act as chemical messengers (Burgen et al., 1980). Most toxicological studies have focused on the neurotransmitters listed in Table 5, because considerable background information on these neurotransmitters is already available. Nearly every class of neuron contains some marker enzyme (Table 5), and these have been useful in studies in which attempts have been made to identify neurotransmitter specific cells and in the determination of the regional distribution of neurotransmitter systems.

6.5.1 Synthesis/degradation

Many neurotoxic compounds have been reported to alter steady-state levels of neurotransmitters, but it is difficult to draw functional inferences from such data since the steady-state levels of neurotransmitters can be influenced via multiple mechanisms (e.g., rate of synthesis, rate of release, rate of degradation). More informative data are obtained by examination of the turnover rates, reflecting the metabolic half-life of the neurotransmitter (Costa, 1970). Turnover of 5-HT, after disulfiram treatment, was examined by observing the accumulation of 5-HT following administration of pargyline (Minegishi et al., 1979). It has been speculated that carbon disulfide acts by altering brain catecholamine concentrations.

Table 5. Enzyme markers for neurotransmitter specific cells

Neurotransmitter	Marker enzyme	Receptor types
acetylcholine	choline acetyltransferase	mucarinic, nicotinic
dopamine	tyrosine hydroxylase	DA_1 and DA_2
noradrenaline	dopamine-β-hydroxylase	$\alpha_1, \alpha_2, \beta_1, \beta_2$ adrenoreceptors
GABA (γ-aminobutyric acid)	glutamate decarboxylase	$GABA_A$ and $GABA_B$ (strychnine-insensitive; picrotoxin-sensitive)
glycine	unknown	strychnine-senstive
serotonin	l-amino acid decarboxylase	$5 HT_1$, $5 HT_2$

Carbon disulfide increased DA and decreased NE by inhibiting dopamine β-hydroxylase, the enzyme responsible for converting dopamine (DA) into norepinephrine (NE) (McKenna & DiStefano, 1975). Manganese is known to inhibit DA formation by blocking tyrosine hydroxylase in the striatum (Bonilla, 1980) and many acute effects of organophosphorus compounds are related to inhibition of AChE activity (O'Brien, 1976). Soon after their introduction, the inhibition of AChE was accepted as a mechanism for the acute toxic effects of organophosphorus insecticides (DuBois et al., 1949). However, this mechanism does not account for the delayed neurotoxicity seen after organophosphate poisoning (Abou-Donia & Preissig, 1976; Abou-Donia, 1981).

Interference with axonal transport may also disrupt neurotransmitter function by altering the availability of neurotransmitter enzymes or by decreasing the transport of peptide precursors. The transport of materials along axons is bidirectional: anterograde and retrograde. Anterograde transport conveys materials from cell body to axon and terminals at slow (1 - 3 mm per day) and fast (410 mm per day) rates (Ochs, 1972; Hoffman & Lasek, 1975). The former contains the bulk of axoplasmic proteins (notably of neurofilaments and neurotubules) and the latter, membrane and other components. Retrograde transport, a system that conveys materials at rapid rates (300 mm per day) may also be affected early in toxic axonopathies. Retrograde transport may be a critical factor in the toxicity resulting from exposure to various compounds.

6.5.2 Transport/release

Neurotransmitters or their precursors can rapidly concentrate in nerve endings through specific high-affinity uptake systems associated with each transmitter-specific class of neurons (Iverson, 1971). The high-affinity, Na^+-dependent transport mechanisms are specific to nerve cells and can be distinguished from the ubiquitous low-affinity transport systems that concentrate a large variety of amino acids, sugars, and nucleosides, or their precursors. High-affinity uptake phenomena may be studied in brain homogenates, brain minces, or synaptosomal preparations. Lead (Silbergeld & Goldberg, 1975), the insecticide chlordecone (Chang-tsui & Ho, 1979), and erythrosin B (Lafferman & Silbergeld, 1979) have been reported to interfere with neurotransmitter uptake processes. However, a variety of nonspecific events may influence apparent uptake, so caution must be exercised in interpreting results of these studies. For example, the effects of erythrosin B on uptake mechanisms were reported to be non-specific (Mailman et al., 1980).

The release of neurotransmitters from synaptic endings occurs through an exocytotic process that is triggered by an influx of calcium ions on depolarization of the nerve endings (Cotman et al., 1976). Neurotransmitter release can be measured by preloading nerve endings with labelled neurotransmitters, exposing tissue slices or synaptosomal fractions maintained on filter beds to calcium ions, and measuring the appearance of labelled or unlabelled compounds in the supernatant medium (Bondy & Harrington, 1979). Heavy metals such as lead have been reported to interfere with calcium-dependent neurotransmitter release (Bondy et al., 1979; Ramsay et al., 1980), and manganese has been reported to block transmitter release (Kirpekar et al., 1970; Balnave & Gage, 1973; Kostial et al., 1974), possibly by blocking inward Ca^{2+} current (Baker et al., 1971). Again, caution must be used in comparing the results from different assay systems.

6.5.3 Binding

Binding of neurotransmitters to specific membrane receptors is the first step in a complex series of events initiated in the post-synaptic cell. Such binding interactions are reversible, stereospecific, nonenzymatic, have equilibria with low dissociation contants, and involve configurational recognition (Yamamura et al, 1981). Studies on receptor binding have been made possible by the availability of specific radioactive analogues of neurotransmitters. In general, the most potent binding ligands are the pharmacological antagonists or agonists of a given neurotransmitter, rather than the transmitter itself. Kinetic characteristics of binding and receptor density are estimated by incubating receptor-enriched membranes with radioactive ligands. Excess ligands, not bound to membranes, can be removed by filtration or centrifugation. Non-specific binding of the labelled compound is estimated by repeating the incubation in the presence of a high concentration (10^{-4} to 10^{-6} mol) of an unlabelled analogue. The solubility of ligands either in lipids or in water has to be considered when interpreting results of ligand-binding studies. This method is relatively simple and has been suggested as a useful screening procedure for the detection of neurotoxic compounds (Damstra & Bondy, 1980, 1982). If properly employed, such analyses can provide valuable information. However, interpretation of the data can be complicated by the often low degree of specificity of the ligand and the location of the receptor, which may be pre- or post-synaptic or on non-neuronal glial elements. Furthermore, for many neurotransmitters, several subtypes of receptors exist and may produce different effects on the post-synaptic membrane. Functional extrapolations from neurotransmitter binding studies, therefore, should be made with caution.

Receptor binding techniques have only recently been applied to neurotoxicological studies. However, in a short time, many compounds have been reported to increase or decrease estimates of receptor density. Acrylamide (Bondy et al., 1981), chlordecone (Seth et al., 1981), lead and mercury (Bondy & Agrawal, 1980), and cadmium (Hedlund et al., 1979) have all been reported to alter putative neurotransmitter receptors.

6.5.4 Ion channels

Many neuronal functions are regulated by ion channels. The Na^+ channel is responsible for depolarizing the membrane, and K^+ channels are responsible for repolarizing the membrane. Maintenance of appropriate Na^+ and K^+ concentrations requires the classical Na^+/K^+ ATPase. Disturbed functioning of these ion channels or disturbance of ATP availability can severely disturb neuronal functioning. Several naturally-occurring toxins affect Na^+ channels (Hille, 1976; Ritchie, 1979; Catterall, 1977). Tetrodotoxin and saxitoxin inactivate the channel at nanomolar concentrations and can be used as probes for measuring channel density or isolation of channel polypeptides (Agnew et al., 1978). Batrachotoxin and veratridine bind the channels and produce persistent activation by preventing channel inactivation (Albuquerque & Daly, 1976). Peptide toxins, such as scorpion toxin (Couraud et al., 1978), exhibit either voltage sensitive or insensitive binding to the extracellular surface of the Na^+ channel (Catterall, 1977). Several potassium channels probably exist in neurons (Reichardt & Kelly, 1983), but purification and characterization of these channels has lagged behind that of the Na^+ channel. However, a scorpion toxin that exibited K^+ channel affinity has been described (Carbone et al., 1982).

Na^+/K^+-ATPase consists of 2 polypeptide chains. The smaller polypeptide is a glycoprotein (Carilli et al., 1982). The larger polypeptide binds ATP internally and ouabain externally. Hormones and neurotransmitters such as catecholamines regulate the ATPase (Clausen & Flatman, 1977), and neurotoxicants could alter neuronal functioning by disturbing this control of ionic gradients. Desaiah et al. (1980) have reported inhibition of Na^+/K^+-ATPase and decreased ouabain binding to synaptosomes after treatment of mice with the insecticide chlordecone. The evaluation of ion balance and their control will probably be used increasingly in neurotoxicology.

For the most part, transmitter release is regulated by Ca^{2+} entry through a Ca^{2+}-selective channels. Depolarization, neurotransmitters, and hormones regulate Ca^{2+}-selective channel (Reichardt & Kelly, 1983). Nerve terminals contain several Ca^{2+}-calmodulin-dependent protein kinases and a Ca^{2+}-phospholipid activated kinase, each of which has a distinct set of protein substrates. Cytoplasmic Ca^{2+} binds calmodulin and other Ca^{2+} binding proteins, which directly or indirectly activate other enzymes via their Ca^{2+}-dependent kinases. How such activation facilitates exocytosis is not known, but presumably the phosphorylation state of synapsin I, a phosphoprotein present primarily in nerve terminals and associated with synaptic vesicles, is believed to regulate transmitter vesicle release (Dolphin & Greengard, 1981).

Changes in Ca^{2+} concentration induced by neurotoxicants could have significant consequences for neuronal function. Cytoplasmic Ca^{2+} stimulates not only exocytosis, but also glucogenolysis and mitochondrial respiration (Landowne & Ritchie, 1976), endocytosis (Ceccarelli & Hurlbut, 1980), and neurotransmitter synthesis (Collier & Ilson, 1977). Even though many of these events are homeostatic responses to transmitter utilization, neurotoxic disruption of calcium influx or sequestering could produce disturbances not restricted to neurotransmitter release.

Few neurotoxic compounds have been investigated for their influence on calcium channels. Manganese is reported to block neurotransmitter release by blocking inward Ca^{2+} current (Kirpekar et al., 1970), and other heavy metals have been reported to interfere with calcium-mediated neurotransmitter release (Bondy et al., 1979; Ramsay et al., 1980). Similar effects of heavy metals were also observed for the Na^+-Ca^{2+} exchange system. Ion channels and Na^+-Ca^{2+} probes may be a valuable screening approach for some types of neurotoxic compounds.

6.5.5 Cyclic nucleotides

Nerve terminal function and the effects of neurotransmitters are often regulated by cyclic nucleotides. Binding of agonists to receptors on the nerve membrane can result in activation of second messenger systems. Activation of different receptors results in specific changes in cyclic AMP and cyclic GMP levels and consequent alterations in protein kinases. It is thought that on phosphorylation, conformational changes occur in membrane proteins that may change ion permeabilities. Thus, the responsiveness of the nervous system to some toxic agents can also be measured by determining changes in the activities of adenylate cyclase, cyclic nucleotides, and protein phosphorylation. For example, lead has been shown to inhibit cerebellar adenylate cyclase (Nathanson & Bloom, 1975) and dopamine-sensitive adenylate cyclase in the striatum (Wilson, 1982). Various pesticides cause increases in the levels of cyclic nucleotides in brain tissue (Aldridge et al., 1978). For example, tri-o-cresyl phosphate enhanced Ca^{2+}-calmodulin-dependent in vivo phosphorylation of proteins in chicken brain (Patton et al., 1983).

6.5.6 Summary of nerve terminal function

The analysis of synaptic function and neurotransmitter metabolism is reasonably complex, and it should be borne in mind that disturbance at many levels of neuronal organization will ultimately alter synaptic function. However, examination of the nerve terminal is an excellent approach for the initial study of toxic chemicals. However, it is important to recognize the dynamic nature of the nerve terminal and to remain alert to the possibility of false positives.

6.6 Energy Metabolism

Nervous tissue, and brain tissue in particular, require disproportionately large amounts of energy to sustain the translocation of ions important for electrical activity and to maintain the highly-active biosynthetic machinery of the tissue. Since neural tissue has only limited stores of energy (e.g., glycogen and creatine phosphate), glucose availability and enzymes critical for energy production are vital to neuronal functioning. A number of neurotoxic chemicals have been shown to interfere with glucose and energy metabolism in both the central and peripheral nervous system. These include methylmercury (Bull & Lutkenhoff, 1975), hexachlorophene (Cammer & Moore, 1972), organotin compounds (Lock, 1976), and alcohol (Merkuryva et al., 1980). Glycolytic enzymes have been shown to be inhibited by alcohol (Merkuryva et al., 1980) and by chemicals known to cause distal axonopathy, e.g., acrylamide (Howland et al., 1980) carbon disulfide, and methyl-n-butyl ketone (Sabri et al., 1979).

Active brain areas have a higher rate of glucose consumption than less active regions. The brain regional metabolic activity is determined by the ^{14}C-2-deoxyglucose method (2-DG) of Sokoloff et al. (1977). This method is based on the use of 2-deoxy-D-^{14}C-glucose as a tracer for the exchange of glucose between the plasma and the blood and its phosphorylation by hexokinase. The product, 2-deoxyglucose-6-phosphate (2-DG-P), is trapped in the tissue and its accumulation in the various regions of the brain might be a measure of the glucose use and neuronal activity. The method provides an index of the in vivo glucose metabolic activity of brain regions and has been used in experimental animals to determine which brain regions are depressed or activated during acute Soman intoxication (McDonough et al., 1983).

Metabolic compartmentalization in nerve tissue could provide an additional tool in toxicological studies. It is well established that neurons mainly use glucose in their energy metabolism, while glia use substrates other than glucose (Hertz, 1981). Thus, it may be possible to differentiate between the toxicological effects of chemical substances on neuronal and glial populations in vitro or in vivo.

6.7 Biochemical Correlates of Axonal Degeneration

A relatively large class of neurotoxic agents is known to produce axonal degeneration (Griffin & Price, 1980; Sabri & Spencer, 1980; Thomas, 1980). Some, such as acrylamide and organophosphorus compounds, produce the distal to proximal "dying back" pattern of degeneration, while others, such as β,β-iminodipropionitrile, lead to proximal to distal degeneration. Since many of these compounds produce Wallerian degeneration, biochemical correlates of Wallerian degeneration have been suggested as toxicological indices (Dewar & Moffett, 1979). These authors tabulated the chemical changes in peripheral nerves that occurred during degeneration and suggested that β-gluocorinadase and β-galactosidase might be good indices of toxicity. Acrylamide, methylmercury, and dimethyl sulfoxide were shown to increase these lysosomal enzymes (Dewar & Moffett, 1979). The use of lysosomal enzymes involves relatively simple procedures and might, therefore, be appropriate for the initiation of a biochemical screen.

Disturbance of axoplasmic transport has been suggested as an alternative approach to detecting compounds producing axonal degeneration. Several substances, e.g., organophosphates (Reichart & About-Donia, 1980) and acrylamide (Pleasure et al., 1969) disrupt axonal transport. However, these methods are more difficult, more expensive, and more time-consuming than the lysosomal enzyme assays.

6.8 Neuroendocrine Assessments

The number of toxic compounds being recognized for their neuroendocrine actions is increasing. Hormonal balance results from the integrated action of the hypothalamus, pituitary, and endocrine target organ. Each site is susceptible to disruption by environmental toxic agents. This disruption may result from the direct interaction of the toxic agent with the endocrine organ, pituitary, or hypothalamus. Alternatively, neuroendocrine dysfunction may occur because of a disturbance in the regulation and/or modulatory elements of the complex neuroendocrine feedback systems. Any such disturbances would ultimately modify anterior pituitary secretions. Thus, the analysis of blood levels is the most appropriate starting point (section 6.8.2.1).

6.8.1 Anterior pituitary hormones

The main effector organ in the neuroendocrine system is the pituitary. This "master gland" consists of an anterior adenohypophysis, and a posterior neurohypophysis. Based on histological, immunocytochemical, and electron microscopic examination, the following cell types are differentiated in the anterior pituitary (Junqueira et al., 1977): follicular cells, which do not contain any secretory granules but form the support stroma of the glandular cells; chromophobe cells, which are undifferentiated, nonsecretory and secretory cells without discernible granules in the light microscope; somatotropic cells, which are acidophilic with immunocytochemically-detectable growth hormone and contain granules of about 350 nm diameter; prolactin cells, which are acidophilic and contain prolactin granules of 600 - 900 nm diameter; gonadotropic cells, which consist of 2 basophilic subgroups: follicle-stimulating hormone secreting and luteinizing-hormone secreting; follicle-stimulating hormone secreting cells, which are large round cells with dense 200 nm diameter granules; luteinizing hormone-containing cells, which are small and contain 200 - 250 nm diameter granules; thyrotropic cells, which are basophilic with thyroid-stimulating hormone granules of 120 - 200 nm diameter; and finally, cortico cells, which are the least abundant of the cell types and contain basophilic granules 100 - 200 nm in diameter.

The glandular cells of the anterior pituitary secrete seven endocrine hormones, of which four act directly on other endocrine glands. Follicle-stimulating hormone (FSH) promotes spermatogenesis in the male testes and facilitates follicular maturation and estrogen secretion in the female ovary. Lutenizing hormone (LH) acts on the male testes to facilitate testosterone secretion from the interstitial cells of Leydig and is a key hormone that promotes follicular rupture (ovulation) in the female ovary. Thyroid-stimulating hormone (TSH) triggers the secretion of thyroxine from the thyroid gland, and adrenocorticotropic hormone (ACTH) causes the adrenal cortex to secrete its products, especially glucocorticoids. The secretion of these tropic, anterior pituitary hormones is in turn regulated by the hormones of the endocrine gland. In most cases, this is a negative feedback regulation. Estrogen decreases the output of pituitary FSH and LH; thyroxine decreases the secretion of TSH; and glucocorticoids reduce the output of ACTH.

The three other anterior pituitary hormones are prolactin (PRL), melanocyte-stimulating hormone (MSH), and growth hormone (GH). A major target for prolactin is the mammary gland, where prolactin promotes milk production. PRL also plays a role in maintaining the ovarian corpus luteum after ovulation. The entire body is a target for GH, which promotes growth and maintainance of cellular integrity. GH facilitates growth, in part, because it increases the transport of amino acids into the cell, where they can be used for protein synthesis. MSH increases the production of melanin by the melanocytes of the skin.

Hypothalamic control of anterior pituitary secretions occurs through the release of hypothalamic-hypophysiotropic hormones (HHH). The hypothalmus secretes these HHH into vessels of the hypothalamic-hypophyseal portal system, by which they are transported to the anterior pituitary. One of the major advances of the last two decades has been the isolation and characterization of these HHH.

6.8.2 Disruption of neuroendocrine function

Disruption of neuroendocrine function can occur at any one or all of the levels of hypothalamic-pituitary-target organ integration. Alternatively, neuroendocrine effects may result from modification of "higher" levels of neuronal processing or from alterations in peripheral metabolism. In the following discussion, approaches will be indicated for the study of each of these possible sites of neurotoxic action.

6.8.2.1 Direct pituitary effects

At the most dramatic level, massive changes in the weight or size of the pituitary, such as occur in the adenohypophysis after large doses of estrogen (Schreiber & Pribyl, 1980) might be seen. However, by far the most accessible method for studying pituitary function relies on the examination of blood levels of pituitary hormones by radioimmunoassay. Furthermore, the analysis of blood-hormone levels is one of the few techniques applicable for screening human populations. A large number of toxic substances have been reported to modify adenohypophyseal secretions. Methallibure and allied substances inhibit thyrotropin (Tulloch et al., 1963), and prolactin (Benson & Zagni, 1965) secretion. Modifications of pituitary hormone secretions have been reported for acrylamide (Uphouse et al., 1982), alcohol (Mendelson et al., 1977), 1,4-DDT (Gellert et al., 1972), and chlordecone (Uphouse et al., 1984). Dimethylsulfoxide may influence adrenal glucocorticoids by elevating pituitary secretions (Allen & Allen, 1975). In spite of the fact that changes in the blood levels of pituitary hormones may be the most sensitive index of neuroendocrine modification by toxic compounds, they have been examined for relatively few compounds. The high sensitivity of this approach results from the fact that the blood levels represent the final consequence of the complex neuroendocrine integration. Regardless of the actual site of modification, neuroendocrine disturbances will usually be revealed in modified levels of circulating hormones. Therefore, such changes, alone, cannot be regarded as evidence of direct neuroendocrine disruption. The major disadvantage of serum-hormone measurements is the responsiveness of the hypothalamic-pituitary axis to a variety of environmental and chemical stimuli. It can be difficult to identify the toxic agent as the causal agent. Because hormones are secreted in a pulsatile manner, single point analyses of serum hormones must be cautiously interpreted. However, even with these limitations, analysis of blood levels of pituitary hormones remains the most appropriate starting point for evaluating potential neuroendocrine toxicity.

Similar analytical methods may be used to investigate the pituitary content of respective pituitary secretions. The pituitary is removed, homogenized, and extracted for use with the appropriate RIA. For most pituitary secretions, neurotoxicologists have not yet studied pituitary tissue directly. However, pituitary endorphins has been reported to be modified by chlordecone (Hong & Ali, 1982).

6.8.2.2 Peripheral target effects

Most anterior pituitary hormones are subject to negative feedback control by peripheral endocrine glands. If the neurotoxic agent modifies peripheral secretions, neuroendocrine changes can result from this altered feedback.

Modifications in the functioning of these endocrine secretions could occur after toxic exposure. Such approaches have been widely applied in the experimental and clinical literature and have shown that a number of compounds alter blood levels of glucocorticoids, thyroxine, estrogen, and testosterones (Chapman, 1983).

Target-tissue effects can also be evaluated by a variety of additional techniques. One of the simplest assessments is the change in the weight, morphology, or biochemistry of the target organ. Various environmental contaminants have been reported to produce such changes. Lesions of the thyroid have been reported after exposure to carbon disulfide (Cavalleri, 1975) and strong magnetic fields (Persinger et al., 1978). Marked changes occur in the adrenals during antimony and lead poisoning (Minkins et al., 1973) and in response to very long chain saturated fatty acids (Powers et al., 1980). Chlordecone causes adrenal, cortical, and medullary hypertrophy (Eroschenko & Wilson, 1975) and alters the epinephrine and norephinephrine content of the adrenal medulla (Baggett et al., 1980). DDT (McBlain et al., 1976) and other chlorinated hydrocarbons (Dicksith & Datta, 1972; Fellegiova et al., 1977), carbon disulfide (Rosewickyi et al., 1973), and cadmium salts (Parizek, 1956; Zylber-Haran et al., 1982) have all been described as having toxic effects on the gonads. Although such changes are not necessarily due to direct neuroendocrine effects, target organ changes can often be a first indication of neuroendocrine changes. In some cases, even relatively gross target organ events have been a first clue towards the mode of action of a neurotoxic agent. For example, the chlorinated pesticides, DDT and chlordecone, modify gonads in a manner reminiscent of the natural steroid, estrogen (Gellert et al., 1972; Eroschenko & Palmiter, 1980; Kupfer & Bulger, 1980). Uterine and/or oviduct weight changes in the immature animal were the first evidence that the pesticides might exert estrogenic action.

6.8.2.3 Disruption of hypothalamic control of pituitary secretions

Hypothalamic control of anterior pituitary secretions includes direct regulation through hypothalamic hypophysiotropic hormones and modulation through neurotransmitters and neurally-active peptides. Evaluation of the effect of a neurotoxic agent on HHH is directly measureable only for the HHH for which antisera are available. For these compounds, it is possible (though difficult) to measure release into the portal blood supply, to evaluate the effects of toxic agents on either amounts or release, and to identify pituitary responsiveness to the hypothalamic factors. Where identified hormones are not available, hypothalamic extracts may still be used with in vitro pituitary responsiveness as a bioassay. Details of such methods can be found in several sources (Burgus & Guillemin, 1970; Oliver et al., 1974). However, the value of such approaches for neurotoxicology has yet to be tested. Such methods will be of greatest value in testing hypotheses regarding the mechanism of action of known neuroendocrine toxic agents. They are not recommended for initial screens.

Biochemical changes in the hypothalamus can also be used as indices of potential neuroendocrine disruption. Such hypothalamic effects of neurotoxic compounds have received much less attention than brain areas such as the striatum, cortex, or cerebellum. Methods for studying the hypothalamus are the same as those used for other brain areas. However, the hypothalamic neurons that regulate pituitary function receive numerous synaptic inputs, both conventional and from putative neurotransmitters. Consequently, the neuroendocrine significance of changes in hypothalamic neurotransmitters and neuropeptides is usually only inferential. However, any disruption of hypothalamic biochemistry has the potential to alter neuroendocrine function. When combined with more direct measurements of neuroendocrine function, such studies are very important. There have been a few reports of biochemical changes in the hypothalamus and/or pituitary, correlated with neuroendocrine toxicity. One approach has been to examine the effects of toxic compounds on hormone-mediated changes. Administration of estrogens is followed by hypothalamic ascorbic acid depletion (Schreiber et al., 1982) and by increases in polyphenol oxidase (ceruloplasmin) activity in the hypothalamus and the blood (Schreiber & Pribyl, 1980). This can be inhibited by the simultaneous administration of silver nitrate. Disulfiram (tetraethylthiuram disulfide) inhibits the reaction of the adenohypophysis (Schreiber et al., 1979). Disulfiram also inhibits dopamine-β-hydroxylase (Szmigielski, 1975) and lowers the blood-prolactin level (Cavalleri et al., 1978). The effect of disulfirams on prolactin may be due to a "sparing of dopamine" through inhibition of dopamine-β-hydroxylase.

Hypothalamic peptides have been studied most extensively after chlordecone treatment. Long-term exposure to the pesticide reduced hypothalamic β-endorphin levels under conditions where substance P, neurotensin, and met-enkephalin were unchanged (Ali et al., 1982).

6.8.2.4 Other sites of action

For many neurotoxic agents, there may be no identifiable effects on neuroendocrine function, but it may be altered through the indirect effects of the toxic compound. Such interruption could occur via modification of neural integration leading to an altered response of the organism to environmental challenge. Detection of such integrative action and its relevance to neuroendocrine function might include treatment with the toxic agent followed by environmental, pharmacological, or hormonal challenges known to produce a neuroendocrine response. Several toxic agents have been reported to produce behavioural changes, such as stress-induced analgesia, and these undoubtedly involve some aspect of neuroendocrine function. CNS opiate systems are important components of the CNS response to stress and studies of peripheral and brain endorphins and encephalins are potentially relevant to such disturbances. For example, neonatal treatment with chlordecone dissolved in dimethyl sulfoxide produces an elevated corticosterone response to footshock (Rosecrans et al., 1982), and long-term exposure of female rats to chlordecone has been reported to decrease hypothalamic β-endorphin levels (Ali et al., 1982).

A toxic agent could also indirectly affect neuroendocrine function by altering the peripheral metabolism of endocrine secretions. Such metabolic differences could indirectly influence CNS function. However, hormone transformation and the formation of active metabolites occurs in the CNS so that metabolic disturbances may even have a direct effect on CNS functioning. Many metabolic variables have been reported to change after treatment with a toxic agent. Aromatization of testosterone to estrogen, an important step in the metabolism of estrogen, took place in the brain of animals (Gallard et al., 1978). Its inhibition by aminoglutethimide or other blockers of aromatization (Morali et al., 1977) markedly altered the sexual behaviour of experimental animals. Aminoglutethimide also inhibited total adrenal steroidogenesis as well as gonadal steroidogenesis and thyroid function (Schreiber et al., 1969). The transformation of thyroxine to the more active metabolite triiodothyroinine was inhibited by a series of toxic substances such as ethanol (Shimizu et al., 1978), propylthiouracil (Leonard & Rosenberg, 1980), iopanoic acid (Kaplan, 1980), and sodium salicylate (Chopra et al., 1980). Since the monodeiodination of thryoxine to triiodothyronine also takes place in the adenohypophysis, these factors may be an important component of neuroendocrine reactions to neurotoxic substances. There is evidence that demonstrates that the direct dopaminergic effect of estrogen on the pituitary may require conversion of estrogen to catechol estrogen (Paul et al., 1980). Such conversion occurs not only in the pituitary, but also in the hypothalamus and cerebral cortex and may mediate some of the effects of estrogen on the CNS. Study of this enzyme promises to be important for future research, especially for the investigation of estrogen-like toxic agents.

A final way in which the toxic agent might disrupt neuroendocrine function is by altering the peripheral metabolism of the endocrine secretions within liver tissue. Although beyond the scope of this publication, several neurotoxic agents (chlordecone, dieldrin, heptachlor, lindane, p,p'-DDE, and toxaphene) stimulate the metabolism of estrone by liver microsomal enzymes (Welch et al., 1971). Biochemical approaches for identifying these metabolic disturbances are the same as those discussed in other sections. However, the precise metabolic end-point should be carefully chosen, when inferences are to be made about neuroendocrine function.

6.8.3 Sex differences

Because neurotoxic agents may produce changes in neuroendocrine function and, since males and females differ with regard to a variety of metabolic variables, a valuable approach to any neurotoxicological investigation is the comparison of the toxic response in the sexes. Whenever neuroendocrine effects are suspected, sex differences should be a routine aspect of the overall investigation. Sex-related differences have been observed for many environmental compounds. Often, these result from the influence of gonadal hormones on the metabolism of the compound. Hormonal influences on the biotransformation and toxicity of DDT (Durham et al., 1956) and several organophosphates (Murphy & DuBois, 1958; DuBois & Puchala, 1961) have been demonstrated. Parathion is an organophosphate insecticide that exerts its toxicity through its active metabolite paraoxon phosphate. Agrawal et al. (1982) have recently shown that the sex difference in AChE inhibition after parathion treatment was not evident with paraoxon treatment. This suggests that the sex difference was in the rate of metabolism to the toxic product. The female's increased sensitivity to amobarbital (Castro & Gillette, 1967) may also be due to sex differences in hepatic metabolism. Sex differences have also been reported for the rate of disposition of chlordiazepoxide (Greenblatt et al., 1977; Roberts et al., 1979) and for the toxic effects of ethylmorphine, aniline, p-nitroanisole (Nicholas & Barron, 1932; Holck et al., 1937; Quinn et al., 1958) and polychlorinated hydrocarbons (Lamartiniere et al., 1979).

6.9 Recommendations for Future Research

Several biochemical and neuroendocrine approaches are available that have not yet been applied to the study of neurotoxic compounds. These have the advantage of increasing the sensitivity of the biochemical approach and furthering understanding of the ways in which compounds disrupt nervous system function. For example, some enzymes involved in neurotransmitter synthesis have been purified and used for the production of specific antibodies (John et al., 1973). It is now possible to use immunological titration to determine whether changes in enzyme activity result from activity alterations or variations in the amount of enzyme protein.

Identification of direct pituitary modification can be accomplished by preparation of anterior pituitary cell cultures and the measurement of hormone release in response to hypothalamic releasing factors, neurotransmitters, or suspect toxic compounds. The pituitary cells are removed, dispersed, and agitated with collagenase. After resuspension in medium, the cells are plated and used for examination. Under such culture conditions, pituitary cells respond to releasing factors and neurotransmitter regulation (Enjalbert et al., 1978; Drouin & Labrie, 1981). Thus, it is possible to determine whether the toxic agent modifies the responsiveness of the pituitary to hypothalamic control. By comparing the effects of the toxic agent in vivo with those in vitro, direct versus indirect effects of the compound can be identified.

Furthermore, for suspect steroid-like compounds, direct evaluation of receptor interactions is possible. Steroid receptors modify their target tissue by binding to intracellular receptors. Measurement of intracellular steroid receptors involves the preparation of a high speed cytosol (180 000 g) fraction from the appropriate target tissue. Identification of binding is accomplished by incubating the cytosol in vitro in the presence of radioactively-labelled hormone. Bound label is removed from unbound by a variety of techniques distinct for the particular receptor of interest. Specific binding is assessed by incubating the labelled hormone in the presence of excess unlabelled hormone as competitor. Specific binding refers to bound molecules that are removed in the presence of this unlabelled competitor. When a neurotoxic agent is suspected of interacting with hormone receptors, the toxic agent may be substituted for the unlabelled competitor and its ability to compete for binding determined. This procedure has demonstrated competition by both chlordecone (Palmiter & Mulvihill, 1978) and o,p'-DDT (Kupfer & Bulger, 1976) for the estradiol cytosol receptor in the uterus. Using an estradiol exchange method, investigators have shown that these pesticides produce translocation of the estradiol receptor to the nucleus (Hammond et al., 1979). Employment of the exchange method necessitates the in vivo treatment of the organism with the toxic agent. Nuclei and cytosol are prepared from the target tissue and incubated in vitro with the radioactively-labelled hormone. Since a major movement of cytosol receptors into the nucleus occurs only after binding to the hormone, the presence of the receptor in the nucleus after exposure to the toxic agent suggests direct binding of the toxic agent to the steroid cytosol receptor.

Modifications of the procedures described for neurotransmitter receptor binding are used in the measurement of membrane receptors. However, no neurotoxic agents have yet been tested for their ability to modify these hormone receptors. For both intracellular and extracellular hormone receptors, most studies have been on peripheral tissues. However, the brain and the pituitary contain receptors for a variety of steroid and peptide hormones, and these offer a number of targets for disruption by environmental compounds. Such analyses have great potential for future studies of neurotoxic compounds. However, they will usually be applied for the investigation of mechanisms of action rather than as screens for neurotoxic compounds.

Finally, hypothalamic regulation of pituitary function should receive further emphasis. Neurotransmitters also regulate pituitary secretions via neurotransmitter receptors of the pituitary gland. The potential for a direct modification of these receptor interactions by neurotoxic compounds is only just being realized. The most thoroughly described pituitary neurotransmitter receptor is that of dopamine, which regulates the inhibition of prolactin release by dopamine. Steroid hormones, such as estrogen, by conversion to catechol estrogens, increase prolactin secretion by direct interaction with the pituitary dopamine receptors (Gudelsky et al., 1981; Fishman, 1982). Neuroleptic drugs elevate prolactin secretion by antagonistic action on pituitary dopamine receptors (Horowski & Graf, 1979; Besser et al., 1980).

7. CONCLUSIONS AND RECOMMENDATIONS

There is ample evidence of real and potential hazards of environmental chemicals for nervous system function. Changes or disturbances in central nervous function, many times manifest by vague complaints and alterations in behaviour, reflect on the quality of life; however, they have not yet received attention. Neurotoxicological assessment is therefore an important area for toxicological research.

It has become evident, particularly in the last decade, that low-level exposure to certain toxic agents can produce deleterious neural effects that may be discovered only when appropriate procedures are used. While there are still episodes of large-scale poisoning, concern has shifted to the more subtle deficits that reduce functioning of the nervous system in less obvious, but still important ways, so that intelligence, memory, emotion, and other complex neural functions are affected.

Information on neurobehaviour, neurochemistry, neurophysiology, neuroendocrinology, and neuropathology is vital for understanding the mechanisms of neurotoxicity. One of the major objectives of a multifaceted approach to toxicological studies is to understand effects across all levels of neural organization. Such a multifaceted approach is necessary for confirmation that the nervous system is the target organ for the effect. Interdisciplinary studies are also necessary to understand the significance of any behavioural changes observed and thus, to aid in extrapolation to human beings by providing specific neurotoxic profiles. Concomitant measurements at different levels of neural organization can improve the validity of results.

The following recommendations are made on the basis of the information contained in this book:

1. Health personnel should take into account the possible role of exposure to chemicals whenever a patient presents with any neurobehavioural complaint.

2. Neurotoxicological testing should be an essential consideration in any profile developed by the agencies responsible for the control of toxic chemicals.

3. In the determination of the potential of a chemical to produce neurotoxic effects, a multidisciplinary strategy should be used.

4. Priority should be given to obtaining clinical and epidemiological data when exposure occurs to chemicals suspected of being neurotoxic.

5. Test development in preclinical neurotoxicology has evolved to the point where interlaboratory validation of procedures using prototypic neurotoxic agents could be attempted.

REFERENCES

ABOU-DONIA, M.B. (1981) Organophosphorus ester-induced delayed neurotoxicity. Ann. Rev. Pharmacol. Toxicol., 21: 511-548.

ABOU-DONIA, M.B. & PREISSIG, S.H. (1976) Delayed neurotoxicity of leptophos: toxic effects on the nervous system of hens. Toxicol. appl. Pharmacol., 35: 269-282.

ABOU-DONIA, M.G., JENSEN, D.N., & LAPADULA, D.M. (1983) Neurologic manifestations of tri-o-cresyl phosphate delayed neurotoxicity in cats. Neurobehav. Toxicol. Teratol., 5: 431-442.

AGNEW, W.S., LEVINSON, S.R., BRABSON, J.S., & RAFTERY, M.A. (1978) Purification of the tetrodotoxin-binding component associated with the voltage-sensitive sodium channel from Electrophorus electricus electroplax membranes. Proc. Natl Acad. Sci. (USA), 75: 2606-2610.

AGRAWAL, A.K., SQUIBB, R.E., & BONDY, S.C. (1981) The effects of acrylamide treatment upon the dopamine receptor. Toxicol. appl. Pharmacol., 58: 89-99.

AGRAWAL, D.K., MISRA, D., AGARWAL, S., SETH, P.K., & KOHLI, J.D. (1982) Influence of sex hormones on parathion toxicity in rats: antiacetylcholinesterase activity of parathion and paraoxon in plasma, erythrocytes, and brain. J. Toxicol. environ. Health, 9: 451-459.

ALBURQUERQUE, E.X. & DALY, J.W. (1976) Steroidal alkaloid toxins and ion transport in electrogenic membranes. In: Cuatracasas, P., ed. The specificity of animal, bacterial, and plant toxins, London, Chapman and Hall, pp. 297-338.

ALDER, S. & ZBINDEN, G. (1977) Methods for the evaluation of physical, neuromuscular, and behavioral development in rats in early postnatal life. In: Newbert, D., Merber, H.J., & Kwasigroch, T.E., ed. Methods in prenatal toxicology, Stuttgart, George Thiene, pp. 175-185.

ALDRIDGE, W.M., CLOTHIER, B., FORSHAW, P., JOHNSON, M.K., PARKER, V.H., PRICE, R.J., SKILLETER, D.N., VERSCHOYLE, P.D., & STEVENS, C. (1978) The effect of DDT and pyrethroids cismethrin and decamethrin on the acetylcholine and cyclic nucliotide content of rat brain. Biochem. Pharmacol., 27: 1703-1706.

ALEU, F.P., KATZMAN, R., & TERRY, R.D. (1963) Fine structures and electrolyte analyses of cerebral oedema induced by alkyl tin intoxication. J. Neuropathol. exp. Neurol., 22: 403-413.

ALEXANDER, B.K., BEYERSTEIN, B.L., HADAWAY, P.F., & COAMBS, R.B. (1981) Effect of early and later colony housing on oral ingestion of morphine in rats. Pharmacol. Biochem. Behav., 15: 571-576.

ALFANO, D.P. & PETIT, T.L. (1981) Behavioral effects of postnatal lead exposure. Possible relationship to hippocampal dysfunction. Behav. neural Biol., 32: 319-333.

ALI, S.F., HONG, J.S., WILSON, W.E., LAMB, J.C., MOORE, J.A., MASON, G.A., & BONDY, S.C. (1982) Subchronic dietary exposure of rats to chlordecone (kepone) modifies levels of hypothalamic beta-endorphin. Neurotoxicology, 3: 119-124.

ALLEN, J.P. & ALLEN, C.F. (1975) The effect of dimethyl sulfoxide on hypothalamic-pituitary-adrenal functions in the rat. Ann. NY Acad. Sci., 243: 325-336.

ALTMAN, J. & SUDARSHAN, K. (1975) Postnatal development of locomotion in the laboratory rat. Anim. Behav., 23: 896-920.

AMIN-ZAKI, L., MAJEED, M.A., ELHASSANI, S.B., CLARKSON, T.W., GREENWOOD, M.R., & DOHERTY, R.A. (1979) Prenatal methylmercury poisoning: clinical observations over five years. J. Dis. Child, 133: 172-177.

ANDRIANOV, V.V., ZAKHAROV, N.C., & FADEEV, JU.A. (1977) Microionophoretic analysis of chemical properties of cortical units in freely moving animals. Physiol. J. (USSR), 63(4): 602-605.

ANGELL, F. & WEISS, B. (1982) Operant behavior of rats exposed to lead before or after weaning. Toxicol. appl. Pharmacol., 63: 62-71.

ANGER, W.K. (1984) Neurobehavioral testing of chemicals: impact on recommended standards. Neurobehav. Toxicol. Teratol., 6(2): 147-153.

ANGER, W.K. & JOHNSON, B.L. (1985) Chemicals affecting behavior. In: O'Donoghue, J.L., ed. Neurotoxicity of industrial and commercial chemicals, Boca Raton, Florida, CRC Press.

ANGER, W.K. & SETYES, J.V. (1979) Effects of oral and intramuscular carbaryl administration on repeated chain acquisition in monkeys. J. Toxicol. environ. Health, 5: 793-808.

ANNAU, W. (1975) The comparative effects of carbon monoxide and hypoxia on behaviour. In: Weiss, B. & Laties, V.G., ed. Behavioural toxicology, New York, Plenum Press, pp. 105-127.

ANOKHIN, P.K. (1935) [Problem of center and periphery in contemporary physiology of nervous system.] In: Anokhin, P.K., ed. [Problem of centre and periphery in physiology of nervous activity], Gorkiy, Gorkiy Publishing House, pp. 9-71 (in Russian).

ANOKHIN, P.K. (1964) [Comparative electrophysical analysis of alterations of laility of the cortical potential components in postnatal ontogenesis.] Fiziol. Zh. SSSR, 50: 773-778 (in Russian).

ANOKHIN, P.K. (1968) [Biology and neurophysiology of the conditioned reflex,] Moscow, Meditsina, pp. 547 (in Russian).

ANOKHIN, P.K. (1974) The functional system as a basis of the physiological architecture of the behavioural act. In: Anokhin, P.K., ed. Biology and neurophysiology of the conditioned reflex and its role in adaptive behaviour, New York, Pergamon Press, pp. 190-254.

APFELBACH, R. & DELGADO, J.M.R. (1974) Social hierarchy in monkeys (Macaca mulatta) modified by chlordiazepoxide hydrochloride. Neuropharmacology, 13: 11-20.

APPEL, S.H. & DAY, E.D. (1976) Cellular and subcellular fractionation. In: Seigel, G.L., Albers, R.W., Katzman, R., & Agranoff, B.W., ed. Basic neurochemistry, Boston, Toronto, Little, Brown and Company, pp. 34-57.

ARBUKHANAOVA, M.S. (1981) Metabolism of glutamic acid in the cerebral mitochondria during cooling disease. In: Mitochondria: the mechanisms of conjugation and regulation, Puschino, p. 76.

ASABAYEV, CH., BONCHKOVSKAYA, T.YU., & ZHEGALLO, I.G. (1972) [A study of the reaction of the animal nervous system to the effect of low-strength electromagnetic fields.] In: [Labour hygiene and the biological effect of radio frequency electromagnetic fields,] Moscow, pp. 48-49 (in Russian).

AVROVA, N.F. (1971) Brain ganglioside patterns of vertebrates. J. Neurochem., 18: 667-674.

BAENNINGER, L.P. (1966) The reliability of dominance orders in rats. Anim. Behav., 14: 367-371.

BAGGETT, J.MCC., THURESON-KLEIN, A., & KLEIN, R.L. (1980) Effects of chlordecone on the adrenal medulla of the rat. Toxicol. appl. Pharmacol., 52: 313-322.

BAKER, P.F., HODGKIN, A.L., & RIDGWAY, E.B. (1971) Depolarization and calcium entry in giant squid axons. J. Physiol., 218: 709-775.

BAKIR, F., DAMLUJI, S.F., AMIN-ZAKI, L., MURTADHA, M., KHALIDI, A., AL-RAWL, N.Y., TIKRITI, S., DHARIR, H.I., CLARKSON, T.W., SMITH, J.C., & DOHERTY, R.A. (1973) Methylmercury poisoning in Iraq: an inter-university report. Science, 181: 230-241.

BALNAVE, R.J. & GAGE, P.W. (1973) The inhibitory effect of manganese on transmitter release at the neuromuscular junctions of the toad. Br. J. Pharmacol., 47: 339-352.

BANCROFT, J.D. & STEVENS, A. (1977) Theory and practice of histological techniques, New York, Churchill Livingston.

BARKER, J.L. & MCKELVY, J.F., ed. (1983) Current methods in cellular neurobiology: electrophysiological and optical recording techniques, New York, John Wiley and Sons, Vol. 3.

BARRETT, R.J., LEITH, N.J., & RAY, O.S. (1973) A behavioral and pharmacological analysis of variables mediating active avoidance behaviour in rats. J. comp. Physiol. Psychol., 82: 489-500.

BARRETT, R.J., LEITH, N.J., & RAY, O.S. (1974) An analysis of the facilitation of avoidance acquisition produced by delta-amphetamine and scopolamine. Behav. Biol., 11: 189-203.

BASAR, E. (1980) EEG-brain dynamics. In: Relation between EEG and brain-evoked potentials, Amsterdam, Oxford, New York, Elsevier Science Publishers.

BAUMGARTNER, G., GAWEL, M.J., KAESER, H.E., PALLIS, C.A., CLIFFORD, F.R., SCHAUMBURG, H.H., THOMAS, P.K., & WADIA, N.H. (1979) Neurotoxicity of halogenated hydroxyquinolines: clinical analysis of cases reported outside Japan. J. Neurol. Neurosurg. Psychiatr., 42: 1073-1083.

BEARD, R.R. & GRANDSTAFF, N. (1975) Carbon monoxide and human function. In: Weiss, B. & Laties, V., ed. Behavioural toxicology, New York, Plenum Press, pp. 1-26.

BECK, E.C., DUSTMAN, R.E., & LEWIS, E.G. (1975) The use of the averaged evoked potential in the evaluation of central nervous system disorders. Int. J. Neurol., 9: 211-232.

BENESOVA, O., HORVATH, M., & MIKISKA, A. (1956) [Assessment of the depth and duration of narcosis according to the electrophysiological characteristics of the cerebral cortex.] Physiol. bohemoslov., 5: 188-194 (in German).

BENNETT, S. & BOWERS, D. (1976) An introduction to multivariate techniques for social and behavioral sciences, New York, Halsted Press.

BENSON, C.K. & ZAGNI, P.A. (1965) The effect of 1-alpha-methylallylthiocarbamyl-2-methylthiocarbamylhydrazine (ICI 33828) on lactation in the rat. J. Endocr., 32: 275-285.

BERGER, H. (1929) [On the electroencephalogram in man.] Arch. Psychiat. Nervenkr., 87: 527-550 (in German).

BERNARD, C. (1927) An introduction to the study of experimental medicine, New York, MacMillan Inc., p. 127.

BESSER, G.M., DELITALA, G., GROSSMAN, A., STUBBS, W.A., & YEO, T. (1980) Chlorpromazine, haloperidol, metoclopramide, and domperidone release prolactin through dopamine antagonism at low concentrations but paradoxically inhibit prolactin release at high concentrations. Br. J. Pharmacol., 71: 569-573.

BHAGAT, B. & WHEELER, M. (1973) Effect of amphetamine on the swimming endurance of rats. Neuropharmacology, 12: 1161-1165.

BIGNAMI, G., ROSIC, N., MICHALEK, H., MILOSEVIC, M., & GATTI, G.L. (1975) Behavioral toxicity of anticholinesterase agents: methodological, neurochemical and neuropsychological aspects. In: Weiss, B. & Laties, V.G., ed. Behavioral toxicology, New York, Plenum Press, pp. 155-215.

BLACKWOOD, W., MCMENEMEY, W.H., MEYER, A., NORMAN, R.M., & RUSSELL, D.S. (1971) Greenfield's neuropathology, London, Edward Arnold Publishing, Ltd.

BLOOM, A.S., STOOTZ, C.G., & DIERINGER, T. (1983) Pyrethroid effects on operant responding and feeding. Neurobehav. Toxicol. Teratol., 5: 321-324.

BOER, G.J. (1974) A microassay for arylamidase activity. Anal. Biochem., 59: 410-411.

BOKINA, A.I., EKSLER, N.D., SEMENENKO, A.D., & MERKURYVA, R.V. (1976) Investigation of the mechanism of action of atmospheric pollutants on the central nervous system and comparative evaluation of methods of study. Environ. Health Perspect., 13: 37-42.

BOKINS, A.I., KAN, T.M., BEREZINA, O.V., & PINIGINA, I.A. (1979) [Study of complex forms of animal behavior in a hygenic evaluation of toxic substances.] Gig. i Sanit., 7: 49-51 (in Russian).

BONASHEVSKAYA, T.I., SHAMARIN, A.A., KESAREV, V.S., & YURASOVA, O.I. (1983) [Morphological criteria and a system of indexes for the evaluation of neurotoxic effects produced by environmental chemical factors (on the basis of a carbon monoxide model).] Gig. i Sanit., 10: 31-33 (in Russian, with English summary).

BONDY, S.C. & AGRAWAL, A.K. (1980) The inhibition of cerebral high affinity receptor sites by lead and mercury compounds. Arch. Toxicol., 46: 249-256.

BONDY, S.C. & HARRINGTON, M.L. (1979) Calcium-dependent release of putative neurotransmitters in the chick visual system. Neuroscience, 4: 1521-1527.

BONDY, S.C., HARRINGTON, M.L., ANDERSON, C.L., & PRASAD, K.N. (1979) Low concentration of an organic lead compound alters transport and release of putative neurotransmitters. Toxicol. Lett., 3: 35-41.

BONDY, S.C., TILSON, H.A., & AGRAWAL, A.K. (1981) Neurotransmitter receptors in brains of acrylamide-treated rats. II. Effects of extended exposure to acrylamide. Pharmacol. Biochem. Behav., 14: 533-537.

BONILLA, E. (1980) L-tyrosine hydroxylase activity in the rat brain after chronic oral administration of manganese chloride. Neurobehav. Toxicol., 2: 37-41.

BONILLA, E., SALAZAR, E., VILLASMIL, J.J., & VILLALOBOS, R. (1982) The regional distribution of manganese in the normal human brain. Neurochem. Res., 7: 221-227.

BOYES, W.K., JENKINS, D.E., & DYER, R.S. (1985) Chlordimeform produces contrast-dependent changes in visual-evoked potentials in hooded rats. Exp. Neurol., 89: 391-407.

BRACELAND, F.J. (1942) Mental symptoms following carbon disulfide absorption and intoxication. Ann. intern. Med., 16: 246-261.

BRADLEY, P.B. (1958) The central action of certain drugs in relation to the recticular formation of the brain. In: Jasper, H.H., Proctor, L.D., Knighton, R.S., Noshay, W.C., & Costello, R.T., ed. Reticular formation of the brain, Boston, Toronto, Little, Brown and Company, pp. 123-149.

BRADY, K., HERRERA, Y., & ZENICK, H. (1976) Influence of parental lead exposure on subsequent learning ability of offspring. Pharmacol. Biochem. Behav., 3: 561-565.

BRIERLEY, J.B. (1976) Cerebral hypoxia. In: Blackwood, W. & Corsellis, J., ed. Greenfield's neuropathology, London, Edward Arnold Publishing, Ltd., pp. 43-85.

BROWN, A.W., ALDRIDGE, W.N., STREET, B.W., & VERSCHOYLE, R.D. (1979) The behavioural and neuropathological sequelae of intoxication by trimethyltin compounds in the rat. Am. J. Pathol., 97: 59-82.

BUELKE-SAM, J. & KIMMEL, C.A. (1979) Development and standardization of screening methods for behavioral teratology. Teratology, 20: 17-29.

BULL, R.J. & LUTKENHOFF, S.D. (1975) Changes in the metabolic responses of brain tissue to stimulation, in vitro, produced by in vivo administration of methylmercury. Neuropharmacology, 14: 351-359.

BURES, J. & BURESOVA, O. (1979) New methods in memory research. In: Proceedings of the 21st Annual Meeting of the Czechoslovak Psychopharmacological Society, Jesenik Spa, 9-14 January, 1979, pp. 7-12.

BURESOVA, O. & BURES, J. (1982) Capacity of working memory in rats as determined by performance on a radial maze. Behav. Processes, 7: 63-72.

BURGEN, A.S.V., KOSTERLITZ, H.W., & IVERSEN, L.L., ed. (1980) Neuroactive peptides, London, Royal Society.

BURGUS, R. & GUILLEMIN, R. (1970) Chemistry of thyrotropin releasing factor (TRF). In: Meites, J., ed. Hypophysiotropic hormones of the hypothalamus: assays and chemistry, Baltimore, Maryland, Williams and Wilkins Company, pp. 227-241.

BUSHNELL, P.J. & BOWMAN, R.E. (1979) Effects of chronic lead ingestion on social development in infant rhesus monkeys. Neurobehav. Toxicol., 1: 207-219.

BUTCHER, R.E. (1976) Behavioral testing as a method for assessing risk. Environ. Health Perspect., 18: 75-81.

BUTCHER, R.E. & VORHEES, C.V. (1979) A preliminary test battery for the investigation of the behavioral teratology of selected psychotropic drugs. Neurobehav. Toxicol., 1(Suppl. 1): 207-212.

CABE, P.A. & TILSON, H.A. (1978) Hind limb extensor response: a method for assessing motor dysfunction in rats. Pharmacol. Biochem. Behav., 9: 133-136.

CAMMER, W. (1980) Toxic demyelination: biochemical studies and hypothetical mechanisms. In: Spencer, P.S. & Schaumburg, H.H., ed. Experimental and clinical neurotoxicity, Baltimore, Maryland, Williams and Wilkins Company, pp. 239-256.

CAMMER, W. & MOORE, C.L. (1972) The effect of hexachlorophene on the respiration of brain and liver mitochondria. Biochem. biophys. Res. Comm., 46: 1887-1894.

CANNON, S.B., VEAZEY, J.M., Jr, JACKSON, R.S., BURSE, V.W., HAYES, C., STRAUB, W.E., LANDRIGAM, P.J., & LIDDLE, J.A. (1978) Epidemic kepone poisoning in chemical workers. Am. J. Epidemiol., 17: 529.

CARBONE, E., WANKE, E., PRESTIPINO, G., POSSANI, L.D., & MAELICKE, A. (1982) Selective blockage of voltage-dependent K^+ channels by a novel scorpion toxin. Nature (Lond.), 296: 90-91.

CARILLI, C.T., FARLEY, R.A., PERLMAN, D.M., & GANTHEY, L.C. (1982) The active site structure of Na^+- and K^+-stimulated ATPase. J. biol. Chem., 257: 5601-5606.

CASARETT, L.J. (1975) Toxicologic evaluation. In: Casarett, L.J. & Doull, J., ed. Toxicology: the basic science of poisons, New York, MacMillan Inc., pp. 11-25.

CASTRO, J.A. & GILLETTE, J.R. (1967) Species and sex differences in the kinetic constants for the N-demethylation of ethyl-morphine by liver microsomes. Biochem. biophys. Res. Comm., 28: 426-430.

CATTERALL, W.A. (1977) Activation of the action potential Na$^+$ ionophore by neurotoxins. J. biol. Chem., 252: 8669-8676.

CAVALLERI, A. (1975) Serum thyroxine in the early diagnosis of carbon disulfide poisoning. Arch. environ. Health, 30: 85-87.

CAVALLERI, A., POLATTI, F., & BOLIS, P.F. (1978) Acute effects of tetramethylthiuram disulfide on serum levels of hypophyseal hormones in humans. Scand. Work environ. Health, 4: 66-72.

CAVANAGH, J.B. (1964) The significance of the "dying-back" process in experimental and human neurological disease. Int. Rev. exp. Pathol., 3: 219-267.

CAVANAGH, J.B. & CHEN, F.C.-K. (1971) The effects of methyl-mercury-dicyandiamide on the peripheral nerves and spinal cord of rats. Acta neuropathol., 19: 208-215.

CAVANAGH, J.B. & JACOBS, J.M. (1954) Some quantitative aspects of diphtheritic neuropathy. Br. J. exp. Pathol., 45: 309-327.

CAVANAGH, J.B., PASSINGHAM, R.J., & VOGT, J.A. (1964) Staining of sensory and motor nerves in muscles with Sudan Black B. J. Pathol. Bacteriol., 88: 89-92.

CECCARELLI, B. & HURLBUT, W.P. (1980) Ca-dependent recycling of synaptic vesicles at the frog neuromuscular junction. J. cell Biol., 87: 297-303

CHANCE, M.R.A. (1946) Aggregation as a factor influencing the toxicity of sympathomimetic amines in mice. J. Pharmacol. exp. Ther., 87: 214-219.

CHANG, L. (1977) Neurotoxic effects of mercury - a review. Environ. Res., 14: 329-373.

CHANG, L. (1980) Mercury. In: Spencer, P.S. and Schaumburg, H.H., ed. Experimental and clinical neurotoxicology, Baltimore, Maryland, Williams and Wilkins Company, pp. 508-526.

CHANG-TSUI, Y.H. & HO, I.K. (1979) Effects of kepone (chlordecone) on synaptosomal gamma-aminobutryic acid uptake in the mouse. Neurotoxicology, 1: 357-361.

CHAPMAN, R.M. (1983) Gonadal injury resulting from chemotherapy. Am. J. ind. Med., 4: 149-161.

CHIBA, S. & ANDO, K. (1976) Effects of chronic administration of kanamycin on conditioned suppression to auditory stimulus in rats. Jpn. J. Pharmacol., 26: 419-426.

CHO, E.S., SPENCER, P.S., JORTNER, B.S., & SCHAUMBURG, H.H. (1980) A single intravenous injection of doxorubicin (Adriamycin^R) induces sensory neuropathy in rats. Neurotoxicology, 1: 583-591.

CHOPRA, I.J., SOLOMON, D.J., TECO, G.N.C., & NGUYEN, A.H. (1980) Inhibition of hepatic outer ring monodeiodination of thyroxine and 3,3',5'-triiodothyronine by sodium salicylate. Endocrinology, 106: 1728-1734.

CIOMS (1983) Safety requirements for the first use of new drugs and diagnostic agents in man, Geneva, Council for International Organizations of Medical Sciences.

CITOVIC, I.S. (1930) [The procedure of studying the effects of oil products on the organism of animals.] Inst. Work Saf., 1: 92 (in Russian).

CLAUSEN, T. & FLATMAN, J.A. (1977) The effects of catecholamines on Na-K transport and membrane potential in rat soleus muscle. J. Physiol., 270: 383-414.

COLLIER, B. & ILSON, D. (1977) The effect of preganglionic nerve stimulation on the accumulation of certain analogues of choline by a sympathetic ganglion. J. Physiol., 264: 489-509.

COLLINS, R.D. (1982) Illustrated manual of neurologic diagnosis, 2nd ed., Philadelphia, Pennsylvania, J.B. Lippincott Company.

COLOTLA, V.A. (1981) Adjunctive polydipsia as a model of alcoholism. Neurosci. Biobehav. Rev., 5: 335-342.

COLOTLA, A., BAUTISTA, M., LORENZANA-JIMENEZ, M., & RODRIGUEZ, R. (1979) Effects of solvents on schedule-controlled behavior. Neurobehav. Toxicol., 1(Suppl. 1): 113-118.

CONSTANTOPOULOS, G., MCCOMB, R.D., & DECABAN, A. (1976) Neurochemistry of the mucopolysaccharidoses: brain glycosaminoglycans in normal and four types of mucopolysaccharidoses. J. Neurochem., 26: 901-908.

CORY-SLECHTA, D.A. & THOMPSON, T. (1979) Behavioral toxicity of chronic postweaning lead exposure in the rat. Toxicol. appl. Pharmacol., 47: 151-159.

CORY-SLECHTA, D.A., BISSEN, T., YOUNG, M., & THOMPSON, T. (1981) Chronic postweaning lead exposure and response duration performance. Toxicol. appl. Pharmacol., 60: 78-84.

COSTA, A. & MURAD, J.E. (1969) Study of the association between chlorpromazine and analgesics through the method of electrical stimulation of the rabbit dental pulp. Rev. Bras de Pesgnisa Med. Biol., 2: 235-240.

COSTA, E. (1970) Simple neuronal models to estimate turnover rate of noradrenergic transmitters in vivo. In: Costa, E. & Giabocini, E., ed. Advances in biochemical psychopharmacology. II. Biochemistry of simple neuronal models, New York, Raven Press.

COTMAN, C.W. & BARKER, G.A. (1974) The making of a synapse. Rev. Neurosci., 1: 1-62.

COTMAN, C.W., HAYCOCK, J.W., & WHITE, W.F. (1976) Stimulus secretion coupling processes in brain: analysis of noradrenaline and gamma-aminobutyric acid release. J. Physiol., 254: 475-505.

COURAUD, F.C., ROCHAT, H., & LISSITSKY, S. (1978) Binding of scorpion and sea anemone neurotoxins to a common site related to the action potential Na^+ ionophore in neuroblastoma cells. Biochem. biophys. Res. Comm., 83: 1525-1530.

CRANE, A.M. & GOLDMAN, P.S. (1979) An improved method for embedding brain tissue in albumin-gelatin. Stain Technol., 54: 71-75.

CRAPPER, D.R. & DE BONI, U. (1980) Aluminum. In: Spencer, P.S. & Schaumburg, H.H., ed. Experimental and clinical neurotoxicology, Baltimore, Maryland, Williams and Wilkins Company, pp. 326-335.

CUTLER, M.G. (1977) Effects of exposure to lead on social behaviour in the laboratory mouse. Psychopharmacology, 52: 279-282.

DAMSTRA, T. (1978) Environmental chemicals and nervous system dysfunction. Yale J. Biol. Med., 51: 457-468.

DAMSTRA, T. & BONDY, S.C. (1980) The current status and future of biochemical assays for neurotoxicity. In: Spencer, P.S. & Schaumburg, H.H., ed. Experimental and clinical neurotoxicology, Baltimore, Maryland, Williams and Wilkins Company, pp. 820-833.

DAMSTRA, T. & BONDY, S.C. (1982) Neurochemical approaches to the detection of neurotoxicity. In: Mitchell, C.L., ed. Nervous system toxicology, New York, Raven Press, pp. 349-373.

DAUBE, J. (1980) Nerve conduction studies. In: Aminoff, J., ed. Electrodiagnosis in clinical neurology, New York, Churchill Livingstone, pp. 229-264.

DAVIS, M. (1980) Neurochemical modulation of sensory-motor reactivity: acoustic and tactile startle reflexes. Neurosci. Biobehav. Rev., 4: 241-263.

DE JESUS, C.P.V., TOCOFIGHI, J., & SNYDER, D.R. (1978) Sural nerve conduction study in the rat: a new technique for studying experimental neuropathies. Muscle Nerve, 1: 162-167.

DESAIAH, D., GILLILAND, T., HO, I.K., & MEHENDALE, H.M. (1980) Inhibition of mouse brain synaptosomal ATPases and ouabain binding by chlordecone. Toxicol. Lett., 6: 275-285.

DESCLIN, J.C. (1974) Histological evidence supporting the inferior olive as the major source of cerebellar climbing fibres in the rat. Brain Res., 77: 365-384.

DESI, I. (1983) Neurotoxicological investigation of pesticides in animal experiments. Neurobehav. Toxicol. Teratol., 5: 503-515.

DESI, I. & SOS, J. (1962) Central nervous injury by a chemical herbicide. Acta Med. Acad. Sci. Hung., 18: 429-433.

DESI, I. & SOS, J. (1963) Experimental lesions of the central nervous system induced by triorthocresyl phosphate. Acta Physiol. Acad. Sci. Hung., 23: 63-68.

DESI, I., GONCZI, L., SIMON, G., FARKAS, I., & KNEFFEL, Z. (1974) Neurotoxicologic studies of two carbamate pesticides in subacute animal experiments. Toxicol. appl. Pharmacol., 27: 465-476.

DEWAR, A.J. & MOFFETT, B.J. (1979) Biochemical methods for detecting neurotoxicity. A short review. Pharmacol. Ther., 5: 545-562.

DEWAR, A.J., MOFFETT, B.J., & SITTON, M.F. (1977) The effect of anti-inflammatory drugs on retinal dystrophy in the rat. Toxicol. appl. Pharmacol., 42: 65-74.

DEWS, P.B. (1982) Epistemology of screening for behavioral toxicity. In: Mitchell, C.L., ed. Nervous system toxicology, New York, Raven Press, pp. 229-236.

DEWS, P.B. & WENGER, G.R. (1979) Testing for behavioral effects of agents. Neurobehav. Toxicol., 1(Suppl. 1): 119-127.

DIAMOND, S.S. & SLEIGHT, S.D. (1972) Acute and subchronic methylmercury toxicosis in the rat. Toxicol. appl. Pharmacol., 23: 197-207.

DICKSITH, T.S.S. & DATTA, K.K. (1972) Effect of intra-testicular injection of lindane and endrine on the testes of rats. Acta pharmacol., 31: 1-10.

DIETZ, D.D., MCMILLAN, D.E., GRANT, L.D., & KIMMEL, C.A. (1978) Effects of lead on temporally-spaced responding in rats. Drug chem. Toxicol., 1(4): 401-419.

DINGLEDINE, R., ed. (1984) Brain slices, New York, Plenum Press, 442 pp.

DIXON, R.L. (1976) Problems in extrapolating toxicity data for laboratory animals to man. Environ. Health Perspect., 13: 43-50.

DOLPHIN, A.C. & GREENGARD, P. (1981) Neurotransmitter- and neuromodulator-independent alterations in phosphorylation of protein I in slices of rat facial nucleus. J. Neurosci., 1: 192-203.

DRAPER, W.A. (1967) A behavioural study of the home-cage activity of the white rat. Behaviour, 28: 280-306.

DRENTH, H.J., ENSBERG, I.F.G., ROBERTS, D.V., & WILSON, A. (1972) Neuromuscular function in agriculture workers using pesticides. Arch. environ. Health, 25: 395-398.

DROUIN, J. & LABRIE, F. (1981) Interactions between 17 beta-estradiol and progesterone in the control of luteinizing hormone and follicle stimulating hormone release in rat anterior pituitary cells in culture. Endocrinology, 108: 52-57.

DUBOIS, K.P. & PUCHALA, E. (1961) Studies on the sex differences in the toxicity of cholinergic phosphorothioate (26791). Proc. Soc. Exp. Biol. Med., 107: 908-911.

DUBOIS, K.P., DOULL, J., SALERNO, P.R., & COON, J.M. (1949) Studies on the toxicity and mechanisms of action of p-nitrophenyl diethylthionosphosphate (parathion). J. Pharmacol. exp. Ther., 95: 79-91.

DUBOWITZ, V. & BROOKE, M.H. (1973) Muscle biopsy: a modern approach, London, W.B. Saunders.

DUNLOP, D.S., VAN ELDEN, W., & LAJTHA, A. (1975) Optimal conditions for protein synthesis in incubated slices of rat brain. Brain Res., 99: 303-318.

DUNN, A.J. (1975) Intercerebral injections inhibit amino acid incorporation into brain protein. Brain Res., 99: 405-409.

DUNN, A.J. (1977) Measurements of the rate of brain protein synthesis. In: Roberts, S., Lajtha, A., & Gispen, W.H., ed. Mechanisms, regulation, and special function of protein synthesis in the brain, Amsterdam, Oxford, New York, Elsevier Science Publishers, pp. 97-105.

DURHAM, W.F., CUETO, C., Jr, & HAYES, W.J., Jr (1956) Hormonal influence on DDT metabolism in the white rat. Am. J. Physiol., 187: 373-377.

DYCK, P.J., THOMAS, P.K., LAMBERT, E.H., & BUNGE, R. (1984) Peripheral neuropathy, 2nd ed., Philadelphia, Pennsylvania, W.B. Saunders, Vol. 1.

DYER, R.S. (1980) Effects of prenatal and postnatal exposure to carbon monoxide on visually-evoked responses in rats. In: Weiss, B. & Merigan, W., ed. Neurotoxicity of the visual system, New York, Raven Press, pp. 17-33.

DYER, R.S. (1985a) The use of sensory-evoked potentials in toxicology. Fundam. appl. Toxicol., 5: 24-40.

DYER, R.S. (1985b) Neurophysiological measures following exposure to toxic substances. In: Annau, Z., ed. Behavioral toxicology, Baltimore, Maryland, Johns Hopkins.

DYER, R.S. & BOYES, W.K. (1983) Use of neurophysiological challenges for the detection of neurotoxicity. Fed. Proc., 42: 3201-3206.

DYER, R.S., ECCLES, C.U., & ANNAU, Z. (1978) Evoked potential alterations following prenatal methylmercury exposure. Pharmacol. Biochem. Behav., 8: 137-141.

DYER, R.S., SWARTZWELDER, H.S., ECCLES, C.W., & ANNAU, Z. (1979) Hippocampal after discharges and their post-ictal sequelae in rats: a potential tool for assessment of CNS neurotoxicity. Neurobehav. Toxicol., 1: 5-19.

ECKERMAN, D.A., GORDON, W.A., EDWARDS, J.D., MACPHAIL, R.C., & GAGE, M.I. (1980) Effects of scopolamine, pentabarbital, and amphetamine on radial arm maze performance in the rat. Pharmacol. Biochem. Behav., 12: 595-602.

EDWARDS, P.M. & PARKER, V.H. (1977) A simple, sensitive, and objective method for early assessment of acrylamide neuropathy in rats. Toxicol. appl. Pharmacol., 40: 589-591.

EGAN, G.F., LEWIS, S.C., & SCALA, R.A. (1980) Experimental design for animal toxicity studies. In: Spencer, P.S. & Schaumburg, H.H., ed. Experimental and clinical neurotoxicology, Baltimore, Maryland, Williams & Wilkins Company, pp. 708-725.

EICHELMAN, B., HEGSTRAND, L.R., MCMURRAY, T., & KANTAK, K.M. (1981) Cyclic nucleotides and aggressive behaviour. Psychopharmacology of aggression and social behaviour. Pharmacol. Biochem. Behav., 14(Suppl. 1): 7-12.

ELSNER, J., LOOSER, R., & ZBINDEN, G. (1979) Quantitative analysis of rat behaviour patterns in a residential maze. Neurobehav. Toxicol., 1(Suppl. 1): 163-174.

EMSON, P.C. (1983) Chemical neuroanatomy, New York, Raven Press.

ENJALBERT, A., RUBERG, M., & KORDON, C. (1978) Neuroendocrine control of prolactin secretion. In: Robyn, C. & Harter, M., ed. Progress in prolactin physiology and pathology, Amsterdam, Oxford, New York, Elsevier Science Publishers, pp. 83-94.

EROSCHENKO, V.P. & PALMITER, R.D. (1980) Estrogenicity of kepone in birds and mammals. In: McLachlan, J., ed. Estrogens in the environment, Amsterdam, Oxford, New York, Elsevier Science Publishers, pp. 305-325.

EROSCHENKO, V.O. & WILSON, W.O. (1975) Cellular changes in the gonads, liver, and adrenal glands of Japanese quail as affected by the insecticide kepone. Toxicol. appl. Pharmacol., 31: 491-504.

EVANS, H.L. (1978) Behavioral assessment of visual toxicity. Environ. Health Perspect., 26: 53-58.

EVANS, H.L. & WEISS, B. (1978) Behavioral toxicology. In: Blackman, D.E. & Sanger, D.J., ed. Contemporary research in behavioral pharmacology, New York, Plenum Press, pp. 449-487.

EVANS, H.L., LATIES, V.G., & WEISS, B. (1975) Behavioral effects of mercury and methylmercury. Fed. Proc., 34: 1858-1867.

EVANS, H.L., GARMAN, R.H., & WEISS, B. (1977) Methylmercury: exposure duration and regional distribution as determinants of neurotoxicity in non-human primates. Toxicol. appl. Pharmacol., 41: 15-33.

EVANS, W.O. (1962) A comparison of the analgetic potency of some analgesics as measured by the "flinch-jump" procedure. Psychopharmacologia, 3: 51-54.

FADEEV, JU.A. (1980) [Unit activity of the brain cortex in realization of goal-directed behaviour.] Usp. fiziol. nauk., 11(3): 12-46 (in Russian).

FADEEV, JU.A. & ANDRIANOV, V.V. (1971) Methods of registration of neuronal activity in freely-moving animals. Physiol. J. (USSR), 57(8): 1217-1219.

FALCK, B., HILLARP, N.A., THIEME, G., & TORP, A. (1962) Fluorescence of catecholamines and related compounds condensed with formaldehyde. J. Histochem. Cytochem., 10: 348-354.

FALK, J.L. (1970) Readings in behavioral pharmacology, New York, Appleton-Century-Crofts.

FELLEGIOVA, M., ADAMEC, O., & DAHKOVA, A. (1977) [The effect of lindane on the metabolism of testosterone in the rat.] Cs. Hyg., 22: 115-120 (in Slovak).

FERSTER, C.B. & SKINNER, B.F. (1957) Schedules of reinforcement, New York, Appleton-Century-Crofts.

FESTING, M.F. (1979) Properties of inbred strains and outbred stocks, with special reference to toxicity testing. J. environ. Health Toxicol., 5: 53-68.

FILE, S. (1980) The use of social interaction as a method for detecting anxiolytic activity of chlordiarepoxide-like drugs. J. Neurosci. Methods, 2: 219-238.

FINK, G. (1979) Feedback actions of target hormones on hypothalamus and pituitary with special reference to gonadal steroids. Ann. Rev. Physiol., 41: 571-585.

FISHMAN, J. (1982) Catechol estrogens and pituitary function. In: Muldoon, T.G., Mahesh, V.B., & Perez-Ballester, B., ed. Recent advances in fertility research. Part A. Developments in reproductive endocrinology, New York, Alan R. Lyss, pp. 183-189.

FISHMAN, W.H. & BERNFELD, P. (1955) Glucuronidases. In: Colowick, S.P. & Kaplan, N.O., ed. Methods in enzymology, New York, Academic Press, Vol. 1, p. 262.

FITZGERALD, G.J., KAUFMAN, E.E., SOKOLOFF, L., & SHEIN, H.M. (1974) D(-)-beta-hydroxybutyrote dehydrogenase activity in closed cell lines of glial and neuronal origin. J. Neurochem., 22: 1163-1166.

FODOR, G.G., SCHLIPKOTER, H.W., & ZIMMERMAN, M. (1973) The objective study of sleeping behaviour in animals as a test of behaviour toxicity. In: Horvath, M. & Frantik, M., ed. Adverse effects of environmental chemicals and psychotropic drugs, Amsterdam, London, New York, Elsevier Science Publishers, Vol. 1, pp. 115-122.

FOLCH, J., ASCOLI, I., LEES, M., MEATH, J.A., & LEBARON, F.N. (1951) Preparation of lipid extracts from brain tissue. J. biol. Chem., 191: 833-841.

FOWLER, S.C. & PRICE, A.W. (1978) Some effects of chlordiazepoxide and delta-amphetamine on response force during punished responding in rats. Psychopharmacology, 56: 211-215.

FOX, D.A., LOWNDES, H.E., & BIERKAMPER, G.G. (1982) Electrophysiological techniques in neurotoxicology. In: Mitchell, C.L., ed. Nervous system toxicology, New York, Raven Press, pp. 299-335.

FOX, W.M. (1965) Reflex-ontogeny and behavioral development of the mouse. Anim. Behav., 13: 234-241.

FRANKOVA, S. (1970) Behavioral responses of rats to early overnutrition. Nutr. Metab., 12: 228-230.

FRANKOVA, S. (1971) Relationship between nutrition during lactation and maternal behavior of rats. Act. Nerv. Super. (Praha), 13: 1-8.

FRANKOVA, S. (1977) Drug-induced changes in the maternal behavior of rats. Psychopharmacology, 53: 83-87.

FRANTIK, E. (1970) The development of motor disturbances in experimental chronic carbon disulfide intoxication. Med. Lav., 61: 309-313.

FRANTIK, E. & BENES, V. (1984) Central nervous effect and blood level regressions on exposure time paralleled in solvents (toluene, carbon tetrachloride, and chloroform). Act. Nerv. super. (Praha), 26: 131.

FUJIMORI, K., BENET, H., MEHENDALE, H.M., & HO, I.K. (1982) Comparison of brain discrete area distribution of chlordecone and mirex in the mouse. Neurotoxicology, 3: 125-130.

FULLERTON, P.M. (1966) Chronic peripheral neuropathy produced by lead poisoning in guinea-pigs. J. Neuropathol. exp. Neurol., 25: 214-236.

GABE, M. (1976) Histological techniques, New York, Paris, Springer-Verlag, Masson.

GAD, S.C. (1982) Statistical analysis of behavioral toxicology data and studies. Arch. Toxicol., Suppl. 5: 256-266.

GAD, S.C. & WEIL, C.S. (1982) Statistics for toxicologists. In: Hayes, A.W., ed. Principles and methods of toxicology, New York, Raven Press, pp. 270-320.

GALLARD, G.V., PETRO, Z., & RYAN, K.J. (1978) Phylogenetic distribution of aromatase and other androgen-converting enzymes in the central nervous system. Endocrinology, 10: 2283-2290.

GELLER, I., MENDEZ, V., HAMILTON, M., HARTMANN, R.J., & GAUSE, E. (1979) Effects of carbon monoxide on operant behavior of laboratory rats and baboons. Neurobehav. Toxicol., 1(Suppl. 1): 179-184.

GELLERT, R.J., HEINRICHS, W.L., & SWERDLOFF, R.S. (1972) DDT homologues: estrogen-like effects on the vagina, uterus, and pituitary of the rat. Endocrinology, 91: 1095-1100.

GERHART, J.M., HONG. J.S., UPHOUSE, L.L., & TILSON, H.A. (1982) Chlordecone-induced tremor: quantification and pharmacological analysis. Toxicol. appl. Pharmacol., 66(2): 234-243.

GILLIATT, R.W. (1973) Recent advances in the pathophysiology of nerve conduction. In: Desmedt, J.E., ed. New developments in electromyography and clinical neurophysiology, Basel, Karger, Vol. 2, pp. 2-18.

GLATT, A.F., TALAAT, H.N., & KOELLA, W.P. (1979) Testing of peripheral nerve function in chronic experiments with rats. Pharmacol. Ther., 5: 539-543.

GLAUSERT, A.M. (1980) Fixation, dehydration, and embedding of biological specimens, Amsterdam, Oxford, New York, Elsevier Science Publishers.

GLOWINSKI, J. & IVERSEN, L.L. (1966) Regional studies of catecholamines in the rat brain. I. The disposition of 3H-norephinephrine, 3H-dopamine, and 3H-DOPA in various regions of the brain. J. Neurochem., 13: 655-699.

GOLDSTEIN, B.D., LOWNDES, H.E., & CHO, E.S. (1981) Neurotoxicology of vincristine in the cat: electrophysiological studies. Arch. Toxicol., 48: 253-264.

GONCHARUK, V.D. (1981) Alteration of activity of glutamate dehydrogenase in ganglionated neurons of rabbits under acute experimental emotional stress. Bull. exp. Biol. Med., 10: 494-496.

GOOD, P. (1979) Detection of a treatment effect when not all experimental subjects will respond to treatment. Biometrics, 35: 483-489

GORIDIS, C., MASSARELLI, R., SERSENBRENNER, M., & MANDEL, P. (1974) Guanyl cyclase in chick embryo brain cell cultures: evidence of neuronal localization. J. Neurochem., 23: 135-139.

GOYER, R.A. & RHYNE, B.C. (1973) Pathological effects of lead. Int. Rev. exp. Pathol., 12: 1-7.

GRANT, L.D. (1976) Research strategies for behavioral toxicology studies. Environ. Health Perspect., 18: 85-94.

GRAY, E.G. & WHITTAKER, V.P. (1962) The isolation of nerve endings from brain: an electron microscopic study of the cell fragments of homogenation and centrifugation. J. Anat., 96: 79-87.

GREENBLATT, D.J., SHADER, R.I., FRANKE, K.K., MACLAUGHLIN, E.D., RONSIL, G.J., & KOCH-WESER, J. (1977) Kinetics of intravenous chlordiazepoxide: sex differences in drug metabolism. Clin. Pharmacol. Ther., 22: 893-903.

GREENGARD, P. (1979) Cyclic nucleotides, phosphorylated proteins and the neuronal system. Fed. Proc., 38: 2208-2217.

GREGORY, E.H. & PFAFF, D.W. (1971) Development of olfactory-guided behavior in infant rats. Physiol. Behav., 6: 573-576.

GRIFFIN, J.W. & PRICE, D.L. (1980) Proximal axonopathies induced by toxic chemicals. In: Spencer, P.S. & Schaumburg, H.H., ed. Experimental and clinical neurotoxicology, Baltimore, Maryland, Williams and Wilkins Company, pp. 161-178.

GRIFFIN, J.W., PRICE, D.L., KLUTHE, D.O., & GOLDBERG, M.A. (1980) Neurotoxicity of misonidazole in rats. Neuropathol. appl. Neurobiol., 6: 656-666.

GROSS-SELBECK, E. & GROSS-SELBECK, M. (1981) Changes in operant behavior of rats exposed to lead at the accepted no-effect level. Clin. Toxicol., 18: 1247-1256.

GROTA, L.S. & ADER, R. (1969) Continuous recording of maternal behavior in the rat. Anim. Behav., 17: 72-729.

GUDELSKY, G.A., NANSEL, D.D., & PORTER, J.C. (1981) Role of estrogen in the dopaminergic control of prolactin secretion. Endocrinology, 108: 440-444.

HAIDER, S.S., HANSAN, M., & ISLAM, F. (1980) Effect of air pollutant hydrogen sulfide on the levels of total lipids, phospholipids, and cholesterol in different regions of the guinea-pig brain. Ind. J. exp. Biol., 18: 418-420.

HAMMOND, B., KATZENELLENBOGEN, B.S., KRAUTHAMMER, N., & MCCONNEL, J. (1979) Estrogenic activity of the insecticide chlordecone (kepone) and interaction with uterine estrogen receptors. Proc. Natl Acad. Sci. (USA), 76: 6641-6645.

HARPUR, E.S. & D'ARCY, P.F. (1975) The quantification of kanamycin ototoxicity in the rat using conditioned tone discrimination. J. Pharm. Pharmacol., 27: 907-913.

HARRY, G.J. & TILSON, H.A. (1982) Postpartum exposure to triethyltin produces long-term alterations in responsiveness to apomorphine. Neurotoxicology, 3: 64-71.

HASAN, M. & ALI, S.F. (1981) Effects of thallium, nickel, and cobalt administration on the lipid peroxidation in different regions of the rat brain. Toxicol. appl. Pharmacol., 57: 8-13.

HAY, A. (1978) Neurotoxins may go unrecognized. Nature (Lond.), 274: 206.

HAYAT, M.A. (1973) Principles and techniques of electron microscopy, New York, Van Rostrand Reinhold Company, Vols. 1 and 2.

HEDLUND, B., GAMARA, M., & BARTFAI, I. (1979) Inhibition of striatal muscarinic receptors in vivo by cadium. Brain Res., 168: 216-218.

HEISE, G.A. (1983) Toward a behavioural toxicology of learning and memory. In: Zbinden, G., Cuomo, V., Racagni, G., & Weiss, B., ed. Application of behaviour pharmacology and toxicology, New York, Raven Press, pp. 27-38.

HEISE, G.A. & MILAR, C. (1984) Drugs and stimulus control. In: Iverson, S.D. & Snyder, S.H., ed. Handbook of psychopharmacology, New York, Plenum Press, pp. 129-190.

HOFFMAN, H.S. & FLESHLER, M. (1963) Startle reaction: modification by background acoustical stimulation. Science, 141: 928-930.

HERMAN, S.P., KLEIN, R., TALLEY, F.A., & KRIGMAN, M. (1973) An ultrastructural study of methylmercury-induced primary sensory neuropathy in the rat. Lab. Inv., 28: 104-118.

HERTZ, L. (1981) Gamma amino butyric-acid glutamate pathway in glia. 5th European Neuroscience Congress, Liege, Belgium, 14-18 September, 1981. Neurosci. Lett, Suppl. 7: 172.

HETZLER, B.E., HEILBRONNER, R.L., GRIFFIN, J., & GRIFFIN, G. (1981) Acute effects of alcohol on evoked potentials in visual cortex and superior colliculus of the rat. Electroencephalogr. clin. Neurophysiol., 51: 69-79.

HILLE, B. (1976) Gating in sodium channels of nerve. Ann. Rev. Physiol., 38: 139-152.

HINDE, R. (1974) Biological basis of human social behaviour, New York, McGraw Hill, Inc.

HOFFMAN, H.S. & FLESHLER, M. (1963) Startle reaction: modification by background acoustical stimulation. Science, 141: 928-930

HOFFMAN, P.N. & LASEK, R.J. (1975) The slow component of axonal transport. Identification of major structural polypeptides of the axon and their generality among mammalian neurons. J. cell Biol., 66: 351.

HOLCK, H.G.O., MUNIR, A.K., MILLS, L.M., & SMITH, E.L. (1937) Studies upon the sex differences in rats in tolerance to certain barbiturates and to nicotine. J. Pharmacol. exp. Ther., 60: 323-346.

HOLMSTEDT, B. (1959) Pharmacology of organophosphorus cholinesterase inhibitors. Pharmacol. Rev., 11: 567-688.

HONG, J.S. & ALI, S.F. (1982) Chlordecone (kepone) exposure in the neonate selectively alters brain and pituitary endorphin levels in prepuberal and adult rats. Neurotoxicology, 3: 111-118.

HOPF, H.C. & EYSHOLDT, M. (1978) Impaired refractory periods of peripheral sensory nerves in multiple sclerosis. Ann. Neurol., 4: 499-501.

HOROWSKI, D. & GRAF, K.J. (1979) Neuroendocrine effects of neuropsychotropic drugs and their possible influence on toxic reactions in animals and man: the role of dopamine-prolactin system. Arch. Toxicol. Suppl. 2: 93-104.

HORVATH, M., ed. (1973) Adverse effects of environmental chemicals and psychotropic drugs. Quantitative interpretation of functional tests, Amsterdam, Oxford, New York, Elsevier Science Publishers, Vol. 1, 292 pp.

HORVATH, M. & FRANTIK, E. (1973) Quantitative interpretation of experimental toxicological data: the use of reference substances. In: Horvath, M., ed. Adverse effects of environmental chemicals and psychotropic drugs, Amsterdam, Oxford, New York, Elsevier Scientific Publishing Co., Vol. 1, pp. 11-21.

HORVATH, M. & FRANTIK, M., ed. (1976) Adverse effects of environmental chemicals and psychotropic drugs: neurophysiological and behavioural tests, Amsterdam, New York, Oxford, Elsevier, Vol. 2, 334 pp.

HORVATH, M. & FRANTIK, E. (1979) Industrial chemicals and drugs lowering central nervous systems activation level: quantitative assessment of hazard in man and animals. Act. Nerv. super. (Praha), 21: 269-272.

HORVATH, M. & MICHALOVA, C. (1956) Changes of EEG in experimental exposure to carbon disulfide in the light of Vvedenskys theory of parabiosis. Arch. Gewerbepathol., 15: 131-136.

HORVATH, M., FRANTIK, E., & KREKULE, P. (1981) Diazepam impairs alertness and potentiates a similar effect of toluene. Act. Nerv. super. (Praha), 22: 17-19.

HOWLAND, R.D., VYAS, I.L., LOWNDES, H.E., & ARGENTIERI, T.M. (1980) The etiology of toxic peripheral neuropathies: in vitro effects of acrylamide and 2,5-hexanedione on brain enolase and other glycolytic enzymes. Brain Res., 202: 131-142.

HUGHES, J.A. & SPARBER, S.B. (1978) Delta-amphetamine unmasks postnatal consequences of exposure to methylmercury in utero: methods for studying behavioral teratogenesis. Pharmacol. Biochem. Behav., 8: 365-375.

HUNT, V.R., SMITH, M.K., & WORK, D., ed. (1982) Banbury Report II - Environmental factors in human growth and development, New York, Cold Spring Harbor Laboratory.

HUNTER, D. & RUSSELL, D.S. (1954) Focal cerebral and cerebellar atrophy in human subjects due to organic mercury compounds. J. Neurol. Neurosurg. Psychiatr., 17: 235-241.

HUNTER, D., BORNFORD, R., & RUSSELL, D. (1940) Poisoning by methylmercury compounds. Q. S. Med., 9: 193-213.

HUTCHINGS, D.E. (1978) Behavioral teratology: embryopathic and behavioural effects of drugs during pregnancy. In: Gottlieb, G., ed. Studies on the development of behaviour and nervous system: early influences, New York, Academic Press, pp. 7-34.

IRWIN, S. (1968) Comprehensive observational assessment: a systematic quantitative procedure for assessing the behavioral and psychologic state of the mouse. Psychopharmacologia, 13: 222-257.

ISLAM, F., TAYYABA, K., & HASAN, M. (1983) Organophosphate metasystox-induced increment of lipase activity and lipid peroxidation in cerebral hemisphere: diminution of lipids in discrete areas of the brain. Acta pharmacol. toxicol., 53: 121-124.

IVERSEN, L.L. (1971) Role of transmitter uptake mechanisms in synaptic neurotransmission. Br. J. Pharmacol., 44: 571-591.

JACOBWITZ, D.M. (1974) Removal of discrete fresh regions of the rat brain. Brain Res., 80: 111-115.

JOHN, T.H., GEGHMAN, C., & REIS, D.J. (1973) Immunochemical demonstration of increased accumulation of tyrosine hydroxylase protein in sympathetic ganglia and adrenal medulla elicited by reserpine. Proc. Natl Acad. Sci. (USA), 70: 2767-2771.

JOHNSON, B.L. (1980) Electrophysiological methods in neurotoxicity testing. In: Spencer, P.S. & Schaumburg, H.H., ed. Experimental and clinical neurotoxicology, Baltimore, Maryland, Williams and Wilkins Company, pp. 726-742.

JOHNSON, B.L. & ANGER, W.K. (1983) Behavioral toxicology. In: Rom, W.N., ed. Environmental and occupational medicine, Boston, Little Brown and Co., pp. 329-350.

JOHNSON, B.L., ANGER, W.K., SETZIER, J.V., & XINTARAS, C. (1975) The application of a computer-controlled time discrimination performance to problems in behavioral toxicology. In: Weiss, B. & Laties, V.G., ed. Behavioral toxicology, New York, London, Plenum Press, pp. 129-153.

JOHNSON, E.W. (1980) Practical electromyography, Baltimore, Maryland, Williams and Wilkins Company.

JOHNSON, J.E., Jr (1981) Aging and cell structure, New York, Plenum Press, Vol. 1.

JOY, R.M. (1982) Chlorinated hydrocarbon insecticides. In: Ecobichon, D.J. & Joy, R.M., ed. Pesticides and neurological diseases, Boca Raton, Florida, CRC Press, pp. 91-150.

JOY, R.M. (1985) Kindling as a tool in neurotoxicology. Fund. appl. Pharmacol., 5: 41-65.

JOY, R.M., STARK, L.G., PETERSON, S.L., BOWYER, J.T., & ALBERTSON, T.E. (1980) The kindled seizure: production of and modification by dieldrin in rats. Neurobehav. Toxicol., 2: 117-124.

JUNQUEIRA, L.C., CARNEIRO, J., & CONTOPOULOS, A. (1977) Basic Histology, 2nd ed., Los Altos, Lange.

KAPLAN, K.L. (1980) Thyroxine 5'-monodeiodination in rat anterior pituitary homogenates. Endocrinology, 106: 567-576.

KARPOVA, O.B., OBEHOVA, E.L., AVIOVA, N.F., & SCHVARTS, E.G. (1978) [Content and composition of cerebral gangliosides during Down's Syndrome.] Vopros. med. Xhim., 4: 524-527 (in Russian).

KELLEHER, R.T. & MORSE, W.H. (1968) Determinations of the specificity of behavioral effects of drugs. Ergeb. Physiol., 60: 1-56.

KHOLODOV, Ju.A. & SOLOV'EVA, G.R. (1971) [Occasional publication: news on medical equipment manufacture,] fasc. 3, pp. 69-72 (in Russian).

KIMURA, J. (1976) Collision techniques: physiological block of nerve impulses in studies of motor nerve conduction velocity. Neurology, 26: 680-682.

KING, J.A. & VESTAL, B.M. (1974) Visual acuity of peromyscus. J. Mammal., 55: 238-243.

KIRPEKAR, S.M., DIXON, W., & PRATT, J.C. (1970) Inhibitory effect of manganese on norephinephrine release from the splenic nerves of cat. J. Pharmacol. exp. Ther., 174: 72-76.

KLEIN, R., HERMAN, S., BRUBAKER, P.E., & LUCIER, G.W. (1972) A model of acute methylmercury intoxication in rats. Arch. Path., 93: 404-418.

KODAMA, J., FUKUSHIMA, M., & SAKATA, T. (1978) Impaired taste discrimination against quinine following chronic administration of theophylline in rats. Physiol. Behav., 20: 151-155.

KOHLER, W. (1976) The mentality of ages, New York, Liveright, 336 pp.

KONAT, G. & CLAUSEN, J. (1977) Triethyl lead-induced intoxication as an experimental model of hypomyelination. Proc. Int. Soc. Neurochem., 6: 215.

KORNBERG, A. (1955) Lactic dehydrogenase in muscle. In: Colowick, S.P. & Kaplan, N.O., ed. Methods in enzymology, New York, Academic Press, Vol. 1, p. 441.

KOSTIAL, K., LANDEKA, M., & SLAT, B. (1974) Manganese ions and synaptic transmission in the superior cervical ganglion of the cat. Br. J. Pharmacol., 51: 231-235.

KOTLIAREVSKI, L.I. (1951) [Methodology for studying motor conditioned reflexes in some small animals (white rats and guinea-pigs.] Zh. Vyssh. nerv. deyat. imeni, 1(5): 753-761 (in Russian).

KOTLIAREVSKI, L.I. (1957) [Procedure for the investigation of motor-food conditioned reflexes in small animals.] Tr. Inst. Vyssh. nerv. deyat. AN SSR, 3: 23-28 (in Russian).

KRIGMAN, M.R. & HOGAN, E.L. (1974) Effect of lead intoxication on the postnatal growth of the rat nervous system. Environ. Health Perspect., 7: 187-199.

KRINKE, G., SCHAUMBURG, H.H., SPENCER, P.S., SUTER, Y., THOMANN, G., & HESS, R. (1981) Pyridoxine megavitaminosis produces degeneration of peripheral sensory neurons (sensory neuronopathy) in the dog. Neurotoxicology, 2: 13-24.

KRINKE, G., SCHAUMBURG, H.H., SPENCER, P.S., THOMANA, P., & HESS, R. (1979) Clinoquinol and 2,5-hexanedione induce different types of distal axonopathy in the dog. Acta neuropathol., 47: 213.

KRSIAK, M. (1979) Effects of drugs on behavior of aggressive mice. Br. J. Pharmacol., 65: 525-533.

KRUSIUS, T. & FINNE, J. (1977) Structural features of tissue glycoproteins. Fractionation and methylation analysis of gylcopeptides derived from rat brain, kidney, and liver. Eur. J. Biochem., 78: 369-379.

KRYZHANOVSKY, G.N. (1973) Mechanism of action of tetanus toxin. Effect on synaptic processes and some particular features of toxin binding by the nervous tissue. Jaunyn-Schmiedeberg's Arch., 276: 247-270.

KUCZENSKI, R.T. & MANDELL, A.J. (1972) Regulatory properties of soluble and particulate rat brain tyrosine hydroxylase. J. biol. Chem., 247: 3114-3116.

KULKOSKY, P.J., ZELLNER, D.A., HYSON, R.L., & RILEY, A.L. (1980) Ethanol consumption of rats in individual, group, and colonial housing conditions. Physiol. Psychol., 8: 56-60.

KUPFER, D. & BULGER, W.H. (1976) Studies on the mechanism of estrogenic actions of o-p'-DDT; interactions with the estrogen receptor. Pestic. Biochem. Physiol., 6: 561-570.

KUPFER, D. & BULGER, W.H. (1980) Estrogenic properties of DDT and its analogues. In: McLachlan, J., ed. Estrogens in the environment, Amsterdam, Oxford, New York, Elsevier Science Publishers, pp. 239-263.

LAFFERMAN, J.A. & SILBERGELD, E.K. (1979) Erythrosin B inhibition of neurotransmitter accumulation by rat brain homogenate. Science, 206: 363-365.

LAJTHA, A. & MARKS, N. (1971) Protein turnover. In: Lajtha, A., ed. Handbook Neurochemistry, New York, Plenum Press, Vol. 5, pp. 551-629

LAMARTINIERE, C.A., DIERINGER, C.S., & LUCIER, G.W. (1979) Altered ontogeny of glutathione S-transferases by 2,4,5-2',4',5'-hexachlorobiphenyl. Toxicol. appl. Pharmacol., 51: 233-238.

LANDOWNE, D. & RITCHIE, J.M. (1976) On the control of glycogenolysis in mammalian nervous tissue by calcium. J. Physiol., 212: 503-517.

LATIES, V.G. (1982) Contributions of operant conditioning to behavioral toxicology. In: Mitchell, C.L., ed. Nervous system toxicology, New York, Raven Press, pp. 67-80.

LAZAROVA, M., BENDOTTI, C., & SAMANIN, R. (1984) Evidence that the dorsal raphe area is involved in the effect of clonidine against pentylenetetrazol-induced seizures in rats. Naunyn-Schmiedebergs Arch. Pharmacol., 325: 12-16.

LEANDER, J.D. & MACPHAIL, R.C. (1980) Effect of chlordimeform (a formamidine pesticide) on schedule-controlled responding of pigeons. Neurobehav. Toxicol., 2: 315-321.

LEANDER, J.D., MCMILLAN, D.E., & BARLOW, T.S. (1977) Chronic mercuric chloride: behavioural effects in pigeons. Environ. Res., 14: 424-435.

LEHMANN, H.J. & TACKMANN, E. (1974) Neurographic analysis of trains of frequent electrical stimuli in the diagnosis of peripheral nerve disease. Eur. Neurol., 12: 293-308.

LEHRER, G.M. (1974) Measurement of minimal brain dysfunction. In: Xintaras, C., Johnson, B.L., & DeGroot, I., ed. Behavioral toxicology, Cincinnati, Ohio, US Department of Health, Education and Welfare, pp. 450-454 (US DHEW (NIOSH) Publication No. 74-126).

LEONARD, J.L. & ROSENBERG, L.H. (1980) Characterization of essential enzyme sulfhydryl groups of thryoxine 5'deiodinase from rat kidney. Endocrinology, 108: 444-451.

LEVINE, T.E. (1976) Effects of carbon disulfide and FLA-63 on operant behavior in pigeons. J. Pharmacol. exp. Ther., 199: 669-678.

LEWEY, F.H. (1941) Experimental chronic carbon disulfide poisoning in dogs. J. ind. Hyg. Toxicol., 23: 415-535.

LILIENTHAL, H., WINNEKE, G., BROCKHAUS, A., MOLIK, B., & SCHLIPKOTER, H.-W. (1983) Learning set-formation in rhesus monkeys pre- and postnatally exposed to lead. In: Proceedings of the International Conference on Heavy metals in the Environment, Heidelberg, September, 1983, Edinburgh, CEP Consultants, p. 901.

LINDSLEY, D.B. & WICKE, J.D. (1974) The electroencephalogram: autonomous electrical activity in man and animals. In: Thompson, R. & Patterson, M., ed. Bioelectric recording techniques, Part B, New York, Academic Press.

LIPP, J.A. (1968) Cerebral electrical activity following soman administration. Arch. int. Pharmacodyn., 175: 161-169.

LOCK, E.A. (1976) Increase in cerebral fluids in rats after treatment with hexachlorophene or triethyltin. Biochem. Pharmacol., 25: 1455-1458.

LORENZO, A.V. & GERWITZ, M. (1977) Inhibition of ^{14}C-tryptophane transport into brain of lead-exposed neonatal rabbits. Brain Res., 132: 386-392.

LOWITZSCH, K., GOHRING, U., HECKING, E., & KOHLER, H. (1981) Refractory period, sensory conduction velocity, and visual-evoked potentials before and after haemodialysis. J. Neurol. Neurosurg. Psychiatr., 44: 121-128.

LOWNDES, H.E. & BAKER, T. (1976) Studies on drug-induced neuropathies. III. Motor nerve deficit in cats with acrylamide neuropathy. Eur. J. Pharmacol., 35: 177-184.

LOWNDES, H.E., BAKER, T., CHO, E.S., & JORTNER, B.S. (1978a) Position sensitivity of deafferented muscle spindles in experimental acrylamide neuropathy. J. Pharmacol. exp. Ther., 205: 40-48.

LOWNDES, H.E., BAKER, T., MICHAELSON, L.P., & VINCENT-ABLAZEY, M. (1978b) Attenuated dynamic responses of primary endings of muscle spindles: a basis for depressed tendon responses in acrylamide neuropathy. Ann. Neurol., 3: 435-437.

LUKAS, E. (1970) Stimulation electrohypography in experimental toxicology (carbon disulfide neuropathy in rats). Med. Lav., 61: 302-308.

MCBLAIN, W.A., LEWIN, V., & WOLFE, F.H. (1976) Differing estrogenic activities for the enatiomers of o,p'-DDT in immature female rat. Can. J. Physiol., 54: 629-632.

MACDONALD, J.S. & HARBISON, R.D. (1977) Methylmercury induced encephalopathy in mice. Toxicol. appl. Pharmacol., 39: 195-205.

MCDONALD, W.I. (1963) The effects of experimental demyelination on conduction in peripheral nerve. II. Electrophysical observations. Brain, 86: 501-524.

MCDONOUGH, J.H., Jr, HACKLEY, B.E., Jr, CROSS, R., SAMSON, F., & NELSON, S. (1983) Brain regional glucose use during soman-induced seizures. Neurotoxicology, 4: 203-210.

MCKENNA, M.J. & DESTEFANO, V. (1975) A proposed mechanism of action of carbon disulfide on carbon disulfide on dopamine-beta-hydroxylase. Toxicol. appl. Pharmacol., 33: 137.

MCMILLAN, D.E. (1982) Effects of chronic administration of pesticides on schedule-controlled responding by rats and pigeons. In: Chambers, J.E. & Yarborough, J.D., ed. Effects of chronic exposures to pesticides on animal systems, New York, Raven Press, pp. 211-226.

MACPHAIL, R.C. (1982) Studies on the flavour aversions induced by trialkyltin compounds. Neurobehav. Toxicol. Teratol., 4: 225-230.

MACPHAIL, R.C. & LEANDER, J.D. (1980) Flavour aversions induced by chlordimeform. Neurobehav. Toxicol., 2: 363-365.

MACPHAIL, R.C., CROFTON, K.M., & REITER, L.W. (1983) Use of environmental challanges in behavioral toxicology. Fed. Proc., 42: 3196-3200.

MACTUTUS, C.F., UNGER, K.L., & TILSON, H.A. (1982) Neonatal chlordecone exposure impairs early learning and memory in the rat on a multiple measure passive avoidance task. Neurotoxicology, 3: 24-44.

MAGATA, Y. & TSUKADA, W. (1978) Bulk separation of neuronal cell bodies and glial cells from mammalian brain and some of their biochemical properties. Rev. Neurosci., 3: 18-27.

MAILMAN, R.B., FERRIS, R.M., VOGEL, R.A., KILTS, C.D., LIPTOM, M.A., TANG, F.L., SMITH, D.A., MUELLER, R.A., & BREESE, G.R. (1980) Non-specificity of the biochemical actions of erythrosine (Red No. 3): what relation to behavioural changes. Science, 207: 535-537.

MARES, P. & VELISEK, L. (1983) Influence of ethosuximide on metrazol-induced seizures during ontogenesis in rats. Act. Nerv. super (Praha), 25: 292-298.

MARSHALL, J.F. (1975) Increased orientation to sensory stimuli following medial hypothalamic damage in rats. Brain Res., 86: 373-387.

MARSHALL, J.F. & TEITELBAUM, P. (1974) Further analysis of sensory inattention following lateral hypothalamic damage in rats. J. comp. physiol. Psychol., 86: 375-395.

MARSHALL, J.F., TURNER, D.H., & TEITELBAUM, P. (1971) Sensory neglect produced by lateral hypothalamic damage. Science, 174: 523-525.

MARSHALL, J.F., RICHARDSON, J.S., & TEITELBAUM, P. (1974) Nigrostriatal bundle damage and the lateral hypothalamic syndrome. J. comp. Physiol. Psychol., 87: 808-830.

MARSLAND, T.A., GLEES, P., & ERIKSON, L.B. (1954) Modification of Glee's silver impregnation for paraffin sections. J. Neuropathol. exp. Neurol., 13: 587-591.

MASTEROV, A.V. (1974) [Features of the interaction of rats in an electromagnetic field following extinction of conditioned food reactions.] In: [Problems of clinical and experimental medicine,] Moscow, pp. 61-63 (in Russian).

MAURISSEN, J.P.J. (1979) Effects of toxicants on the somatosensory system. Neurobehav. Toxicol., 1(Suppl. 1): 23-32.

MEDVEDEV, B.M. (1975) [The effect of a static electric field on conditioned reflex activity.] Fiziol. Zh., 3: 320-325 (in Russian).

MELLO, N.K. (1975) Behavioral toxicology: a developing discipline. Fed. Proc., 34: 1832-1834.

MENDELL, J.R., SAIDA, K., GANANSIA, M.F., JACKSON, D.B., WEISS, H., GARDIER, R.S., CHRISMAN, C., ALLEN, N., COURI, D., O'NEILL, J., MARKS, B., & HETLAND, L. (1974) Toxic polyneuropathy produced by methyl n-butyl ketone. Science, 185: 787-789.

MENDELSON, J.H., MELLO, N.K., & ELLINGBOE, J. (1977) Effects of acute alcohol intake on pituitary-gonadal hormones in normal human males. J. Pharmacol. exp. Ther., 202: 675-682.

MERIGAN, W.H. (1979) Effects of toxicants on visual systems. Neurobehav. Toxicol., 1: 15-22.

MERIGAN, W.H. (1980) Visual fields and flicker thresholds in methylmercury poisoned monkeys. In: Merigan, W.H. & Weiss, B., ed. Neurotoxicity of the visual system, New York, Raven Press, pp. 149-163.

MERKURYVA, R.V. & BUSHINSKAYA, L.I. (1982) [Metabolism of sialo-containing glycoproteins and lysosomal enzyme activity under neurotropic effect of chemical environmental factors.] Ukranian Biochem. J., 53: 31-35 (in Russian).

MERKURYVA, R.V. & TSAPKOVA, N.N. (1982) Hygienic significance of a system of biochemical criteria for the evaluation of hepatotoxic and neurotoxic effects of some chemical factors in the environment. J. Hyg. Epidemiol. Microbiol. Immunol., 26: 336-341.

MERKURYVA, R.V., BUSHINSKAIA, L.J., AULIKA, B.V., SHATERNIKOVA, J.S., PROTSENKO, S.J., KULYGINA, A.A., & EKSLER, N.D. (1978) The activity of lyosomal and cytoplasmic enzymes under the experimental influence of bisulfide of carbon. Vop. Med. Xhim., 2: 151-156.

MERKURYVA, R.V., KOTOV, A.V., SILOV, V.G., BUSHINSKAIA, L.J., MUCHAMBETOVA, L.KH., & TSAPKOVA, N.N. (1980) Experimental study of biochemical and physiological mechanisms of cerebral activity influenced by alcohol, Nauka, Minsk Publishing House, pp. 93-94.

MEYER, O.A., TILSON, H.A., BYRD, W.C., & RILEY, M.T. (1979) A method for the routine assessment of fore- and hindlimb grip strength of rats and mice. Neurobehav. Toxicol., 1: 233-236.

MICZEK, K.A. & BARRY, H. (1976) Pharmacology of sex and aggression. In: Glick, S.D. & Goldforb, J., ed. Behavioral pharmacology, St. Louis, Missouri, C.V. Mosby Co., pp. 176-257.

MIKISKA, A. (1960) [Determination of the susceptibility to electrical activity of the cerebral motor cortex, and its pharmacological and toxicological applications. I. Methodology, controlled trials and physiological basis.] Arch. Gewerbepathol. Gewerbehyg., 18: 286-299 (in German).

MIKISKOVA, H. & MIKISKA, A. (1962) [A contribution to the application of defensive skin stimulation in the toxicity of substances acting on the CNS. II. Measuring stimulus threshold intensity in guinea-pigs.] Int. Arch. Gewerbepathol. Gewerbehyg., 19: 68-75 (in German).

MIKISKOVA, H. & MIKISKA, A. (1966) Trichloroethanol in trichloroethylene poisoning. Br. J. ind. Med., 23: 116-125.

MIKISKOVA, H. & MIKISKA, A. (1968) Some electrophysiological methods for studying the action of narcotic agents in animals, with special reference to industrial solvents: a review. Br. J. ind. Med., 25: 81-105.

MILLER, D.B. (1983) Neurotoxicity of the pesticidal carbamates. Neurobehav. Toxicol. Teratol., 4: 779-788.

MILLER, E.K. & DAWSON, R.M.C. (1972) Can mitochondria and synaptosomes of guinea-pig brain synthesize phospholipids? Biochem. J., 126: 805-807.

MINEGISHI, A., FUJUMORI, R., SATOH, T., KILAGAWA, H., & YANAURA, S. (1979) Changes in serotonin turnover and the brain sensitivity to barbituates by disulfiram treatment in rats. Res. Comm. Chem. Pathol. Pharmacol., 24: 273-285.

MINKINS, C., CHEKUNOVA, M.P., & LEVINA, E.N. (1973) [Effect of antimony and lead on the adrenal glands and biogenic amines.] Gig. Tr. Prof. Zabol., 17: 21-24 (in Russian).

MITCHELL, C.L. & TILSON, H.A. (1982) Behavioral toxicology in risk assessment: problems and research needs, Boca Raton, Florida, CRC Press, pp. 265-274 (CRC Critical Reviews in Toxicology 10).

MITCHELL, C.L., TILSON, H.A., & CABE, P.A. (1982) Screening for neurobehavioral toxicity: factors to consider. In: Mitchell, C.L., ed. Nervous system toxicology, New York, Raven Press, pp. 237-245.

MIYOSHI, T. & GOTO, I. (1973) Serial in vivo determinations of nerve conduction velocity in rat tails: physiological and pathological changes. Electroencephal. clin. Neurophysiol., 35: 125-131.

MOLINENGO, L. & ORSETTI, M. (1976) Drug action on the "grasping" reflex and on swimming endurance: an attempt to characterize experimentally anti-depressant drugs. Neuropharmacology, 15: 257-260.

MORALI, G., LARSSON, K., & BEYER, C. (1977) Inhibition of testosterone-induced sexual behaviour in the castrated male rat by aromatization blockers. Horm. Behav., 9: 203-213.

MORGANTI, J.B., LOWNE, B.A., SALVATERRA, P., & MASSARO, E.J. (1976) Effects of open-field behaviour of mice exposed to multiple doses of methylmercury. Gen. Pharmacol., 7(1): 41-44.

MUNRO, A.J., JACKSON, R.J., & KORNER, A. (1964) Disaggregation of brain polysomes. Biochem. J., 92: 289-294.

MURPHY, S.D. & DUBOIS, K.P. (1958) The influence of various factors on the enzymatic conversion of organic thiophosphates to anticholinesterase agents. J. Pharmacol. exp. Ther., 124: 194-202.

NARAHASHI, T. (1982) Cellular and molecular mechanisms of action of insecticides: neurophysiological approach. Neurobehav. Toxicol. Teratol., 4: 753-758.

NARAHASHI, T. & HAAS, H.G. (1967) DDT: interaction with nerve membrane conductance changes. Science, 157: 1438-1440.

NARAHASHI, T. & HAAS, H.G. (1968) Interaction with DDT with the components of lobster nerve membrane conductance. J. gen. Physiol., 51: 177-198.

NATHANSON, J.A. & BLOOM, F.E. (1975) Lead-induced inhibition of brain adenylcyclase. Nature (Lond.), 255: 419-420.

NICHOLAS, G.S. & BARRON, D.H. (1932) The use of sodium amytal in the production of anaesthesia in the rat. J. Pharmacol. exp. Ther., 46: 125-129.

NIEDERMEYER, E. & LOPES DA SILVA, F. (1982) Electroencephalography: basic principles, clinical applications, and related fields, Baltimore, Maryland, Munich, Urban Schwartzenberg.

NIOKESARYISKY, A.A. & TUROVSKY, V.S. (1980) N-acetylneuraminic acid content in water-soluble and membranous tissue fractions of various analysers of cerebral cortex. Biochimia, 45: 1829-1932.

NORTON, S. (1973) Amphetamine as a model for hyperactivity in the rat. Physiol. Behav., 11: 181-186.

O'BRIEN, R.D. (1976) Acetylcholinesterase and its inhibition. In: Wilkerson, C.F., ed. Insecticide biochemistry and physiology, New York, Plenum Press, pp. 271-296.

O'CALLAGHAN, J.P., LAVIN, K.L., CHESS, Q., & CLOUET, D.H. (1983) A method for dissection of discrete regions of rat brain following microwave irradiation. Brain Res., 11: 31-42.

O'DONOGHUE, J.L., ed. (1985) Neurotoxicity of industrial and commercial chemicals, Boca Raton, Florida, CRC Press.

OCHOA, J. (1972) Ultrathin longitudinal sections of single myelinated fibres for electron microscopy. J. neurol. Sci., 17: 103.

OCHS, S. (1972) Fast transport of materials in mammalian nerve fibres. Science, 176: 252.

OCHS, S. (1982) Axoplasmic transport and its relation to other nerve functions, New York, John Wiley and Sons.

OHI, G., NISHIGAKI, S., SEKI, H., TAMURA, Y., MIZOGUCHI, I., YAGYA, H., & NAGASHIMA, K. (1978) Tail rotation, an early neurological sign of methylmercury poisoning in the rat. Environ. Res., 16: 353-359.

OLIVER, C., ESKAY, R.L., BEN-JONATHAN, N., & PORTER, J.C. (1974) Distribution and concentration of TRH in rat brain. Endocrinology, 96: 540-546.

OLTON, D.S., BECKER, J.T., & HANDELMANN, G.E. (1979) Hippocampus space, and memory. Behav. Brain Sci., 2: 313-365.

OLTON, D.S., BECKER, J.T., & HANDELMANN, G.E. (1980) Hippocampal function: working memory or cognitive mapping? Physiol. Psychol., 8: 239-246.

OTTO, D.A. (1977) Neurobehavioral toxicology: problems and methods in human research. In: Zenick, H. & Reiter, L.W., ed. Behavioral toxicology: an emerging discipline, Research Triangle Park, North Carolina, US Environmental Protection Agency, pp. 10/1-10/31 (EPA 600/9-77-042).

OTTO, D.A. (1978) Multidisciplinary perspectives in event-related brain potential research. In: Proceedings of the Fourth International Congress on Event-Related Slow Potentials of the Brain, Washington DC, US Environmental Protection Agency (EPA 600/9-77-043).

OTTO, D.A., BENIGNUS, V.A., MULLER, K.E., & BARTON, C.N. (1981) Effects of age and body lead burden on CNS function in young children. I. Slow cortical potentials. Electroencephalogr. clin. Neurophysiol., 52: 229-239.

OVERMANN, S.R. (1977) Behavioral effects of asymptomatic lead exposure during neonatal development in rats. Toxicol. appl. Pharmacol., 41: 459-471.

PADICH, R. & ZENICK, M. (1977) The effects of developmental and/or direct lead exposure on FR behavior in the rat. Pharmacol. Biochem. Behav., 6: 371-375.

PALKOVITS, M. (1973) Isolated removal of hypothalamic or other brain nuclei of the rat. Brain Res., 59: 449-450.

PALMITER, R.D. & MULVIHILL, E.D. (1978) Estrogenic activity of the insecticide kepone on the chick oviduct. Science, 201: 356-358.

PANCHENKO, L.F., DUDCHENKO, A.M., & SHPAKOV, A.A. (1975) The influence of acute hypoxic hypoxia on the activity of rats cerebral cortex: mitochondria enzymes possessing different sensibility to oxygen deficiency. In: Gorky, ed. Biochemistry of hypoxia, pp. 59-64.

PANSKY, B. & ALLEN, D.J. (1980) Review of neuroscience, New York, McMillan Inc.

PARIZEK, J. (1956) Effects of cadmium salts on testicular tissue. Nature (Lond.), 177: 1036-1037.

PARTINGRON, C.R. & DALY, J.W. (1979) Effect of gangliosides on adenylate cyclase activity in rat cerebral cortical membranes. Mol. Pharmacol., 15: 484-491.

PARTRIDGE, W.M. (1976) Inorganic mercury: selective effects on blood-brain barrier transport systems. J. Neurochem., 27: 333-335.

PATTON, S.E., O'CALLAGHAN, J.P., MILLER, D.B., & ABOU-DONIA, M.B. (1983) Effect of oral adminstration of tri-o-cresyl phosphate on in vitro phosphorylation of membrane and cytosolic proteins from chicken brain. J. Neurochem., 41: 897-901.

PAUL, S.M., HOFFMAN, A.R., & AXELROD, A. (1980) Catechol estrogens: synthesis and metabolism in brain and other endocrine tissues. In: Martini, L. & Ganong, W.F., ed. Frontiers in neuroendocrinology, New York, Raven Press, pp. 203-217.

PAVLENKO, S.M. (1975) Methods for the study of the central nervous system in toxicological tests. In: Methods used in the USSR for establishing biologically safe levels of toxic substances, Geneva, World Health Organization, pp. 86-108.

PAVLOV, I.P (1927) Conditioned reflexes, Oxford, Oxford University Press.

PEARSE, A.G.E. (1968) Histochemistry: theoretical and applied, 3rd ed., Baltimore, Maryland, Williams and Wilkins Company.

PEARSON, C.M. & MOSTOFI, F.K. (1973) The striated muscle, Baltimore, Maryland, Williams and Wilkins Company.

PEASE, D.E. (1964) Histological techniques for electron microscopy, 2nd ed., New York, Academic Press.

PERSINGER, M.A., LAFREINIERE, G.P., & CARREY, N.V. (1978) Thyroid morphology and wet organ weight changes in rats exposed to different low intensity 0.5-Hz magnetic fields and pre-experimental caging conditions. Biometeorology, 22: 67-73.

PILCHER, C.W.T. & JONES, S.M. (1981) Social crowding enhances aversiveness of naloxone in rats. Pharmacol. Biochem. Behav., 14: 299-303.

PIRCH, J.H. & RECH, R.H. (1968) Effect of isolation on alpha-methyltyrosine-induced behavioral depression. Life Sci., 7: 173-182.

PLEASURE, D.E., MISHLER, K.C., & ENGEL, W.K. (1969) Axonal transport of proteins in experimental neuropathies. Science, 166: 524-525.

POST, E.M., YANG, M.G., KING, J.A., & SANGER, V.L. (1973) Behavioral changes of young rats force-fed methylmercury chloride. Proc. Soc. Exp. Biol. Med., 143: 1113-1116.

POWERS, J.M., SCHAUMBURG, H.H., JOHNSON, A.E., & RAINE, C.S. (1980) A correlative study of the adrenal cortex in adrenoleukodystrophy: evidence for a fatal intoxication with very long-chain saturated fatty acids. Invest. cell Pathol., 3: 353-376.

PRABHU, V.G. (1972) Amphetamine aggregation effect in mice under conditions of altered microsomal enzymes. Arch. int. Pharmacodyn. Ther., 195: 81-86.

PROKHOROVA, M.J. (1974) Structure and function of phosphornositides and gangliosides of the brain. In: Progress of neurochemistry, Leningrad, Nauka, pp. 61-73.

PRYOR, G.T., UYENO, E.T., TILSON, H.A., & MITCHELL, C.L. (1983) Assessment of chemicals using a battery of neurobehavioral tests: a comparative study. Neurobehav. Toxicol. Teratol., 5: 91-117.

PURPURA, D.P., PENRY, J.K, TOWER, P., WOODBURY, D.M., & WALTER, R. (1972) Experimental models of epilepsy, New York, Raven Press.

QUEVEDO, L., CONCHA, J., MARCHANT, Z., ESKUCHE, W., & MADARIAGA, J. (1980) Nerve accommodation in chronic alcoholic subjects. Pharmacology, 21: 229-232.

QUINN, G.P., AXELROD, J., & BRODIE, B.B. (1958) Species, strain, and sex differences in metabolism of hexobarbitone, amidopyrine, antipyrine, and aniline. Biochem. Pharmacol., 1: 152-159.

RADIN, N.S., BRENHERT, A., ARORA, R.C., SELLINGER, O.Z., & FLANGAS, A.L. (1972) Glial and neuronal localization of cerebroside-metabolizing enzymes. Brain Res., 39: 163-166.

RAFALES, L.S., BORNSCHEIN, R.L., MICHAELSON, A., LOCH, R.K., & BARKER, G.F. (1979) Drug-induced activity in lead-exposed mice. Pharmacol. Biochem. Behav., 10: 95-104.

RAMSAY, R.B., KRIGMAN, M.R., & MORELL, P. (1980) Developmental studies of the uptake of choline, GABA, and dopamine by crude synaptosomal preparations after in vivo or in vitro lead treatment. Brain Res., 187: 383-387.

RAY, O.S. & BARRETT, R.J. (1975) Behavioral, pharmacological, and biochemical analysis of genetic differences in rats. Behav. Biol., 15: 391-417.

REICHARDT, L.F. & KELLY, R.B. (1983) A molecular description of nerve terminal function. Ann. Rev. Biochem., 52: 871-926.

REICHERT, B.L. & ABOU-DONIA, M.B. (1980) Inhibition of fast axoplasmic transport by delayed neurotoxic organophosphorus esters: a possible mode of action. Mol. Pharmacol., 17: 56-60.

REITER, L.W. (1978) Use of activity measures in behavioral toxicology. Environ. Health Perspect., 26: 9-20.

REITER, L.W. (1980) Neurotoxicology - meet the real world. Neurobehav. Toxicol., 2: 73-74.

REITER, L.W. (1983) Chemical exposure and animal activity: utility of the Figure-Eight Maze. In: Hayes, A.H., Schnell, R.C., & Miya, T.S., ed. Developments in the science and practice of toxicology, Amsterdam, Oxford, New York, Elsevier Science Publishers, pp. 78-84.

REITER, L.W. & MACPHAIL, R.C. (1979) Motor activity: a survey of methods with potential use in toxicity testing. Neurobehav. Toxicol., 1(Suppl. 1): 53-66.

REITER, L.W. & MACPHAIL, R.C. (1982) Factors influencing motor activity measurements in neurotoxicology. In: Mitchell, C.L., ed. Nervous system toxicology, New York, Raven Press, pp. 45-65.

REITER, L.W., KIDD, K., HEAVNER, G., & RUPPERT, P. (1980) Behavioral toxicity of acute and subacute exposure to triethyltin in the rat. Neurotoxicology, 2: 97-112.

REUHL, K. & CHANG, L. (1979) Effects of methylmercury on the development of the nervous system: a review. Neurotoxicology, 1: 21-55.

REYNOLDS, G.S. (1958) A primer of operant conditioning, Glenview, Illinois, Scott, Foresman and Co.

RICE, D.C. & GILBERT, S.G. (1982) Early chronic low-level methylmercury poisoning in monkeys impairs spatial vision. Science, 216: 759-761.

RICE, D.C. & WILLES, R.F. (1979) Neonatal low-level lead exposure in monkeys (Macaca fascicularis): effects on two choice non-spatial form discrimination. J. environ. Pathol. Toxicol., 2: 1195-1203.

RICE, D.C., GILBERT, S.G., & WILLES, R.F. (1979) Neonatal low-level lead exposure in monkeys: locomotor activity, schedule-control behavior, and the affects of amphetamine. Toxicol. appl. Pharmacol., 51: 503-513.

RICE, D.F. (1985) Central nervous system effects of perinatal exposure to lead or methylmercury in the monkey. In: Clarkson, T.W. & Nordberg, G., ed. Reproductive developmental toxicity of metals, New York, Plenum Press.

RITCHIE, J.M. (1979) A pharmacological approach to the structure of sodium channels in myelinated axons. Ann. Rev. Neurosci., 2: 341-362.

ROBERTS, D.V. (1977) A longitudinal electromyographic study of six men occupationally exposed to organophosphorus compounds. Int. Arch. occup. environ. Health, 38: 221-229.

ROBERTS, R.K., DESMOND, P.V., WILKINSON, G.R., & SCHENKER, S. (1979) Disposition of chlordiazepoxide: sex differences and effects of oral contraceptives. Clin. Pharmacol. Ther., 25: 826-831.

ROBINS, E., HIRSCH, H.E., & EMMONS, S.S. (1968) Glycosidases in the nervous system. I. Assay, some properties, and distribution of beta-galactosidase, beta-glucoronidase, and beta-glucosidase. J. biol. Chem., 243: 4246-4249.

RODIER, P. (1978) Behavioral teratology. In: Wilson, J.G. & Fraser, F.C., ed. Handbook of teratology, New York, Plenum Press, Vol. 4, pp. 397-428.

ROEDER, R.J. & RUTTER, W.J. (1969) Multiple forms of DNA-dependent RNA polymerase in eukaryotic organisms. Nature (Lond.), 224: 234-236.

ROSE, S.P.R. & SINHA, A.K. (1970) Separation of neuronal and neuropil cell fractions: a modified procedure. Life Sci., 9: 907-912.

ROSECRANS, J.A., HONG, J.S., SQUIBB, R.E., JOHNSON, J.H., WILSON, W.E., & TILSON, H.A. (1982) Effects of perinatal exposure to chlordecone (kepone) on neuroendocrine and neurochemical responsiveness of rats to environmental challenges. Neurotoxicology, 3: 131-142.

ROSEWICKYI, S., STANOSZ, S., & SAMOCHOWIEC, L. (1973) [The effect of protracted exposure to carbon disulfide on the hormonal activity of the ovaries in rats.] Med. Pracy., 24: 133-136 (in Polish).

ROZIER, L., SHIRAKI, H., & GRCEVIC, N., ed. (1977) Neurotoxicology, New York, Raven Press, Vol. 1, 658 pp.

RUDNEV, M., BOKINA, A., ESKLER, N., & NAVAKATIKYAN, M. (1978) The use of evoked potential and behavioural measures in the assessment of environmental insult. In: Proceedings of the Fourth International Congress on Event-Related Slow Potentials of the Brain, Henderson, North Carolina, 4-10 April, 1976 (EPIC IV), Washington DC, US Environmental Protection Agency, pp. 444-447 (EPA 600/9-77-0443).

RUSSELL, R.W., WARBURTON, D.M., & SEGAL, D.S. (1969) Behavioral tolerance during chronic changes in the cholinergic system. Comm. Behav. Biol., 4: 121-128.

RUSAK, B. & ZUCKER, I. (1975) Biological rhythms and animal behavior. Ann. Rev. Psychol., 27: 137-171.

SABRI, M.I. & SPENCER, P.S. (1980) Toxic distal axonopathy: biochemical studies and hypothetical mechanisms. In: Spencer, P.S. & Schaumburg, H.H., ed. Experimental and clinical neurotoxicology, Baltimore, Maryland, Williams and Wilkins Company, pp. 206-219.

SABRI, M.I., MOORE, C.L., & SPENCER, P.S. (1979) Studies on the biochemical basis of distal axonopathies. Inhibition of glycolysis produced by neurotoxic hexacarbon compounds. J. Neurochem., 32: 683-690.

SAKMANN, B. & NEHER, E. (1983) Single channel recording, New York, Plenum Press, 503 pp.

SALVATERRA, P., LOWN, B., MORGANTI, J., & MARSARO, E.J. (1973) Alterations in neurochemical and behavioural parameters in the mouse induced by low doses of methylmercury. Acta pharmacol. toxicol., 33(3): 177-190.

SANTINI, M. (1975) Golgi Centennial Symposium: Perspectives in Neurobiology, New York, Raven Press.

SAVOLAINEN, H. (1983) Trends and prospects in experimental neurotoxicology. Scand. J. Work environ. Health, 9: 214-218.

SAVOLAINEN, H. & JARVISALO, J. (1977) Effects of acute CS_2 intoxication on protein metabolism in rat brain. Chem.-biol. Interact., 17: 51-59.

SAVOLAINEN, H., PFAFFLI, P., TENGEN, M., & VAINO, H. (1977) Biochemical and behavioural effects of inhalation exposure to tetrachloroethylene and dichloromethane. J. Neuropathol. exp. Neurol., 36: 941-949.

SCHALLERT, T., WHISHAW, I.Q., RAMIREZ, V.D., & TEITELBAUM, P. (1978) Compulsive, abnormal walking caused by anticholinergies in akinetic, 6 hydroxydopamine-treated rats. Science, 199: 1461-1463.

SCHAUMBURG, H.H. (1982) Pyridoxine megavitaminosis produces sensory neuropathy in humans. Ann. Neurol., 12: 107-108.

SCHAUMBURG, H.H., SPENCER, P.S., & THOMAS, P.K. (1983) Disorders of peripheral nerves, Philadelphia, Pennsylvania, F.A. Davis.

SCHAUMBURG, H.H., WISNIEWSKI, H., & SPENCER, P.S. (1974) Ultrastructural studies of the dying-back process. I. Peripheral nerve terminal and axon degeneration in systemic acrylamide intoxication. J. Neuropathol. exp. Neurol., 33: 260-284.

SCHECHTER, M.D. & WINTER, J.C. (1971) Effect of mescaline and lysergic acid diethylamide on flicker discrimination in the rat. J. Pharmacol. exp. Ther., 177: 461-467

SCHEUHAMMER, A.M. & CHERIAN, M.G. (1982) The regional distribution of lead in normal rat brain. Neurotoxicology, 3: 85-92.

SCHEVING, L.E., HALBERG, F., & PAULY, J.E., ed. (1974) Chronobiology, Tokyo, Igaku Shoin Ltd.

SCHNAITMAN, C., ERWIN, V.G., & GREENSWALT, J.W. (1967) The submitochondrial localization of monoamine oxidase. An enzymatic marker for the outer membrane of rat liver mitochondria. J. cell Biol., 32: 719-720.

SCHOENFELD, W.N., ed., (1970) The theory of reinforcement schedules, New York, Appleton-Century-Crofts.

SCHOTMAN, P., GIPON, L., JENNEKENS, F.G.I., & GISPEN, W.H. (1978) Polyneuropathies and CNS protein metabolism. III. Changes in protein synthesis induced by acrylamide intoxication. J. Neuropathol. exp. Neurol., 37: 820-837.

SCHREIBER, V. & PRIBYL, T. (1980) Possible role of ceruloplasmin in endocrine regulation. In: Ishü, S., Hirano, T., & Wade, M., ed. Hormones, adaptation, and evolution, Tokyo, Japan Science Society Press/Berlin, Springer-Verlag.

SCHREIBER, V., PRIBYL, T., & JAHODOVA, J. (1982) Inhibition by an ergoline derivative (dopaminergic agonist) of estradiol-induced adenohypophyseal growth and of the decrease in the hypothalamic ascorbic acid (HA) concentration in rats. Physiol. Bohemoslov., 31: 97-100.

SCHREIBER, V., PRIBYL, T., & JAHODOVA, J. (1979) Effect of a dopamine p-hydroxylase inhibitor (disulfiram) on the response of adenohypophysis, serum ceruloplasmin, and hypothalamic ascorbic acid to estradiol treatment. Endoc. Exper. (Bratislava), 13: 131-138.

SCHREIBER, V., ZBUZEK, V., & ZBUZKOVA-KMENTOVA, V. (1969) Reactions of the rat and hamster endocrine system to aminoglutethimide. Physiol. Bohemoslov., 18: 249-261.

SEPPALAINEN, A.M. & LINNOILA, I. (1975) Electrophysiological studies on rabbits in long-term exposure to carbon disulphide. Scand. J. Work environ. Health, 1: 178-183.

SEPPALAINEN, A.M., TOLONEN, M., KARLI, P., HANNINEN, H., & HEINBERG, S. (1972) Neurophysiological findings in chronic carbon disulfide poisoning: a descriptive study. Work Environ. Health, 9: 71-75.

SETH, P.K., AGRAWAL, A.K., & BONDY, S.C. (1981) Biochemical changes in the brain consequent to dietary exposure of developing and mature rats to chlordecone (kepone). Toxicol. appl. Pharmacol., 26: 262-267.

SHANDALA, M.G., RUDNEV, M.I., & NAVAKATIKYAN, M.A. (1980) [Behavioural reactions in experimental hygienic research.] Gig. i Sanit., 6: 43-48 (in Russian).

SHAW, C.M., MOTTET, N.K., & CHEN, W.J. (1980) Effects of methylmercury on the visual system of rhesus macaque (Macaca mulatta). II. Neuropathological findings (with emphasis on vascular lesions in the brain). In: Merigan, W.H. & Weiss, B., ed. Neurotoxicity of the visual system, New York, Raven Press, pp. 123-134.

SHAW, C.M., MOTTET, N.K., BODY, R.L., & LUSCHEI, E.S. (1975) Variability of neuropathological lesions in experimental methylmercury encephalopathy in primates. Am. J. Pathol., 80: 451-470.

SHIBUSAWA, K., YAMAMOTO, T., NISHI, K., ABE, C., & TOMIE, S. (1959) Urinary secretion of TRF in various functional states of the thyroid. Endocrinol. Jpn., 6: 131-136.

SHILJAGINA, N.N. (1971) [Evoked potentials in the projection of sign stimulus during conditional reflex formation in ontogenesis.] Zh. Vyssh. nerv. deyat. imeni, 21: 492-500 (in Russian).

SHIMIZU, T., TAKAISHI, M., & SHISHIBE, Y. (1978) Effect of ethanol on the peripheral metabolism of thyroxine. Endocrinol. Jpn, 25: 201-204.

SHUGALOV, N.P. (1969) Primary and associative evoked responses to optic irritants during various stages of conditioned reflex formation in cats. In: Summary of Reports of the 22nd Meeting on the Problems of Higher Nervous Activity, Ryazan, USSR, p. 268.

SHUMILINA, A.I. (1971) Characteristics of summary electric activity and evoked potentials under motivating stimulation of various biological significance. In: Proceedings of the Sixth All-Union Conference on Electrophysiology of the Central Nervous System, pp. 301-302.

SILBERGELD, E.K. & GOLDBERG, A.M. (1974a) Hyperactivity: a lead-induced behavior disorder. Environ. Health Perspect., 7: 227-232.

SILBERGELD, E.K. & GOLDBERG, A.M. (1974b) Lead-induced behavioral dysfunction: an animal model of hyperactivity. Exp. Neurol., 42: 146-157.

SILBERGELD, E.K. & GOLDBERG, A.M. (1975) Pharmacological and neurochemical investigations of lead-induced hyperactivity. Neuropharmacology, 14: 431-444.

SILBERGELD, E.K., HRUSKA, R.E., MILLER, L.P., & ENG, N. (1980) Effects of lead in vivo and in vitro on GABA energic neurochemistry. J. Neurochem., 34: 1711-1718.

SILVERMAN, A.P. (1965) Ethological and statistical analysis of drug effects on the social behaviour of laboratory rats. Br. J. Pharmacol., 24: 579-590.

SLOANE, S.A., SHEA, S.L., PROCTER, M.M., & DEWSBURY, D. (1978) Visual cliff performance in 10 species of muroid rodents. Anim. Learn. Behav., 6: 244-248.

SNOWDON, C.T. (1973) Learning deficits in lead injected rats. Pharmacol. Biochem. Behav., 1: 599-603.

SNYDER, D.R. & BRAUN, J.J. (1977) Dissociation between behavioral and physiological indices of organomercurial ingestion. Toxicol. appl. Pharmacol., 41: 277-284.

SNYDER, S.H. & INMS, R.B. (1979) Peptide neurotransmitters. Ann. Rev. Biochem., 48: 755-782.

SOBOTKA, T.J., BRODIE, R.E., & COOK, M.P. (1975) Psychophysiologic effects of early lead exposure. Toxicology, 5: 175-191.

SOKOLOFF, L., REIVICH, M., KENNEDY, C., DES ROSIERS, M.H., PATLAK, C.S., PETTIGREW, K.D., SAKURADA, O., & SHINOHARA, M. (1977) The ^{14}C-deoxyglucose method for the measurement of local cerebral glucose utilization: theory, procedure, and normal values in the conscious and anaesthetized albino rat. J. Neurochem., 28: 897-916.

SPENCER, P.S. & BISCHOFF, M.C. (1982) Contemporary neuropathological methods in toxicology. In: Mitchell, C.L., ed. Nervous system toxicology, New York, Raven Press, pp. 259-275.

SPENCER, P.S. & LIEBERMAN, A.R. (1971) Scanning electron microscopy of isolated peripheral nerve fibres. Normal surface structure and alterations proximal to neuromas. Z. Zellforsch. Mikrosk. Anat., 119: 534-551.

SPENCER, P.S. & SCHAUMBURG, H.H. (1980) Experimental and clinical neurotoxicology, Baltimore, Maryland, Williams and Wilkins Company, 929 pp.

SPENCER, P.S. & THOMAS, P.K. (1970) The examination of isolated nerve fibres by light and electron microscopy, with observations on demyelination proximal to neuromas. Acta neuropathol., 16: 177-186.

SPENCER, P.S., BISCHOFF, M., & SCHAUMBURG, H.H. (1980) Neuropathological methods for the detection of neurotoxic disease. In: Spencer, P.S. & Schaumburg, H.H., ed. Experimental and clinical neurotoxicology, Baltimore, Maryland, Williams and Wilkins Company, pp. 743-757.

SPERANSKIJ, S.V. (1965) [Advantages incident to the use of mounting current in analysing the ability of Albino mice to summate subliminal impulses.] Farmakol. i Toksikol., 1: 123-124 (in Russian).

SPYKER, J. (1975) Behavioral teratology and toxicology. In: Weiss, B. & Laties, V.G., ed. Behavioral toxicology, New York, Plenum Press, pp. 311-349.

SQUIBB, R.E. & TILSON, H.A. (1982) Neurobehavioural changes in adult Fisher 344 rats exposed to dietary levels of chlordecone (Kepone^R): a 90-day chronic dosing study. Neurotoxicology, 3: 59-66.

STEBBINS, W.C. (1970) Animal psychophysics: che design and conduct of animal experiments, New York, Appleton-Century-Crofts.

STEEL, R.G.D. & TORRIE, J.H. (1960) Principles and procedures of statistics, New York, McGraw-Hill, pp. 83-347.

STEELE, W.J. & BUSCH, H. (1963) Studies on acidic nuclear proteins of the Walker tumour and liver. Cancer Res., 23: 1153-1157.

STOCKINGER, H.E. (1974) Behavioral toxicology in the development of threshold limit values. In: Xintaras, C., Johnson, B.L., & DeGroot, I., ed. Behavioral toxicology, Cincinnati, Ohio, US Department of Health, Education and Welfare, pp. 18-19 (US DHEW (NIOSH) Publication No. 74-126).

SUDAKOV, K.V. (1982) Functional system theory in physiology. Agressologie, 23: 167-176.

SZMIGIELSKI, A. (1975) Effect of disulfirom and sodium diethyldithiocarbamate on thyroxine and dopamine hydroxylases in rat brain and breast. Pol. J. Pharmacol. Pharm., 27: 153-159.

TAKEUCHI, T. (1968) Pathology of Minamata disease. In: Katsuma, M., ed. Minamata disease. Study Group of Minamata Disease, Japan, Kumamoto University, pp. 141-228.

TAKEUCHI, T., ETO, N., & ETO, K. (1979) Neuropathology of childhood cases of methylmercury poisoning (Minamata disease) with prolonged symptoms with particular reference to the decortication syndrome. Neurotoxicology, 1: 1-20.

TALKE, T., HIRABAGASHI, J., KONDO, R., MATSUMOTO, M., & KOJIMA, K. (1979) Effect of butyrate on glycolipid metabolism of two cell types of rat ascites hepatomes with different ganglioside biosynthesis. J. Biochem., 96: 1139-1402.

TAPPEL, A.L. (1970) Lipid peroxidation damage to cell components. Fed. Proc., 29: 239.

TAYLOR, J.R., SELHORST, J.B., & CALABRESE, V.P. (1980) Chlordecone. In: Spencer, P. & Schaumburg, H.H., ed. Experimental and clinical neurotoxicology, Baltimore, Maryland, Williams and Wilkins Company, pp. 407-421.

THIESSEN, D.D. (1964) Population density and behavior: a review of theoretical and physiological contributions. Texas Rep. Biol. Med., 22: 266-314.

THOMAS, P.K. (1970) The quantitation of nerve biopsy findings. J. neurol. Sci., 11: 285-295.

THOMAS, P.K. (1980) The peripheral nervous system as a target for toxic substances. In: Spencer, P.S. & Schaumburg, H.H., ed. Experimental and clinical neurotoxicity, Baltimore, Maryland, Williams and Wilkins Company, pp. 35-47.

THOMPSON, S.W. (1963) Selected histochemical and histopathological methods, Springfield, Illinois, Charles C. Thomas.

THORNDIKE, E.L. (1932) Reward and punishment in animal learning. Comp. Psychol. Monogr., 39: 8.

TILSON, H.A. & CABE, P.A. (1978) Strategy for the assessment of neurobehavioral consequences of environmental factors. Environ. Health Perspect., 26: 287-299.

TILSON, H.A. & HARRY, G.J. (1982) Behavioral principles for use in behavioral toxicology and pharmacology. In: Mitchell, C.L., ed. Nervous system toxicology, New York, Raven Press, pp. 1-27.

TILSON, H.A. & MITCHELL, C.L. (1984) Neurobehavioral techniques to assess the effects of chemicals on the nervous system. Ann. Rev. Pharmacol. Toxicol., 24: 425-450.

TILSON, H.A. & SQUIBB, R.D. (1982) The effects of acrylamide on the behavioral suppression produced by psychoactive agents. Neurotoxicology, 3: 113-120.

TILSON, H.A., BYRD, N., & RILEY, M. (1979a) Neurobehavioral effects of exposing rats to kepone via the diet. Environ. Health Perspect., 33: 321.

TILSON, H.A., CABE, P.A., ELLINWOOD, E.H., Jr, & GONZALEZ, L.P. (1979b) Effects of carbon disulfide on motor function and responsiveness to delta-amphetamine in rats. Neurobehav. Toxicol., 1: 57-63.

TILSON, H.A., MITCHELL, C.L., & CABE, P.A. (1979c) Screening for neurobehavioral toxicity: the need for and examples of validation of testing procedures. Neurobehav. Toxicol., 1(Suppl. 1): 137-148.

TILSON, H.A., CABE, P.A., & BURNE, T.A. (1980) Behavioral procedures used in the assessment of neurotoxicity. In: Spencer, P.S. & Schaumburg, H.H., ed. Experimental and clinical neurotoxicology, Baltimore, Maryland, Williams and Wilkins Company, pp. 758-766.

TILSON, H.A., MACTUTUS, C.F., MCLAMB, R.L., & BURNE, T.A. (1982a) Characterization of triethyl lead chloride neurotoxicity in adult rats. Neurobehav. Toxicol. Teratol., 4: 671-681.

TILSON, H.A., SQUIBB, R.E., & BURNE, T.A. (1982b) Neurobehavioral effects following a single dose of chlordecone (kepone) administered neonatally to rats. Neurotoxicology, 3: 45-52.

TOLMAN, E.C. (1948) Cognitive maps in rats and men. Psychol. Rev., 55: 189-208.

TOWFIGHI, J., GONATAS, N.K., & MCCREE, L. (1975) Hexachlorophene retinopathy in rats. Lab. Invest., 32: 330-338.

TROPKINA, J.K., SELZNEVA, S.N., & POGODAEV, K.V. (1981) Prenatal influence of hypoxia on metabolic structure of cerebral mitochondria in the oncogenesis with epileptic superactivity. In: Mitochondria: mechanisms of conjugation and regulation, Puscino, p. 39.

TRUEX, R.C. & CARPENTER, M.B. (1983) Human neuroanatomy, 8th ed., Baltimore, Maryland, Williams and Wilkins Company.

TSUJI, S. & FUJIHSIMA H. (1975) Paraplegias: clinical statistics, Fukuoka, Kyushu Rosai Hospital, Department of Orthopedics and Neurology.

TULLOCH, M.L., CROOKS, J., & BROWN, P.S. (1963) Inhibition of thyroid function by a dithiocarbamoylhydrazine. Nature (Lond.), 199: 288-289.

ULRICH, C.E., RINEHART, W., & BRANDT, M. (1979) Evaluation of the chronic inhalation toxicity of a manganese oxide aerosol. III. Pulmonary function, electromyograms, limb tremor, and tissue manganese data. Am. Ind. Hyg. Assoc. J., 40: 349-353.

UPHOUSE, L., NEMEROFF, C.B., MASON, G., PRANGE, A.J., & BONDY, S.C. (1982) Interactions between "handling" and acrylamide on endocrine responses in rats. Neurotoxicology, 3: 121-125.

UPHOUSE, L., MASON, G., & HUNTER, V. (1984) Persistent vaginal estrus and serum hormones after chlordecone (kepone) treatment of adult rats. Toxicol. appl. Pharmacol., 72: 177-186.

US FDA (1978) Nonclinical laboratory studies. Good laboratory practice regulation, Washington DC, US Food and Drug Administration, Department of Health, Education and Welfare (Federal Register 43: 59986-60025).

US NAS (1975) Principles for evaluating chemicals in the environment, Washington DC, National Academy of Science (A Report of the Committee for the Working Conference on Principles of Protocols for Evaluating Chemicals in the Environment).

US NAS/NRC (1970) Evaluating the safety of food chemicals, Washington DC, National Academy of Sciences, National Research Council, Food Protection Committee, Food Nutrition Branch, Division of Biology and Agriculture.

VAN GELDER, G.A. (1978) Lead and the nervous system. In: Oehme, F.W., ed. Toxicity of heavy metals in the environment, Part 1, Basel, New York, Marcel Dekker, Inc., pp. 101-121.

VANDERWOLF, C.H. & LEUNG, L.-W.S. (1983) Hippocampal rhythmic slow activity: a brief history and the effects of entorhinal lesions and phencyclidine. In: Seifert, W., ed.

Neurobiology of the hippocampus, New York, Academic Press, pp. 275-302.

VASAN, N.S. & CHASE, H.P. (1976) Brain glucosaminoglycans (mucopolysaccharides) following intrauterine growth retardation. Biol. Neonate, 28: 196-206.

VEKSLER, M.S. & ARBUKHANOVA, M.S. (1981) Cerebral and spinal cord mitochondria under strenuous physical work. In: Mitochondria: mechanism of conjugation and regulation, Puscino, p. 81.

VERGIEVA, T. & ZAIKOV, H.R. (1981) Behavioral changes in rats with inhalation of styrene. Hig. Zdraveopazvane, 24: 242-247.

VERITY, M.A. (1972) Cation modulation of synaptosomal respiration. J. Neurochem., 19: 1305-1309.

VERITY, M.A., BROWN, W.J., CHEUNG, M., & DZER, G. (1977) Methylmercury inhibition of synaptosomes and brain slices protein synthesis: in vivo and in vitro studies. J. Neurochem., 29: 673-679.

VILA, J. & COLOTLA, V.A. (1981) Some stimulus properties of inhalants: preliminary findings. Neurobehav. Toxicol., 3: 447-480.

VINAR, O., FRANTIK, E., & HORVATH, M. (1981) Subjectively-perceived effects of diazepam, toluene, and their combination. Act. Nerv. super. (Praha), 23: 179-182.

VORHEES, C.V. (1974) Some behavioral effects of maternal hypervitaminosis A in rats. Teratology, 17: 269-273.

VORHEES, C.V. & BUTCHER, R.E. (1982) Behavioral teratogenicity. In: Snell, L., ed. Developmental toxicology, London, Croom Helm Press, pp. 247-298.

VORHEES, C.V., BRUNNER, R.L., MCDANIEL, C.R., & BUTCHER, R.E. (1978) The relationship of gestational age to vitamin A induced postnatal dysfunction. Teratology, 17: 271-276.

WALLMAN, J. (1975) A simple technique using an optomotor response for visual psychophysical measurements in animals. Vision Res., 15: 3-8.

WALSH, J.M., CURLEY, M.D., BURCH, L.S., & KURLANSIK, L. (1982) The behavioral toxicity of a tributyltin ester in the rat. Neurobehav. Toxicol. Teratol., 4: 241-246.

WALSH, R.N. (1980) On the necessity for a shift in emphasis from means-oriented to problems-oriented research in developmental psychobiology. Dev. Psychobiol., 13: 229-231.

WALSH, T.J., MILLER, D.B., & DYER, R.S. (1982b) Trimethyltin, a selective limbic system neurotoxicant, impairs radial-arm maze performance. Neurobehav. Toxicol. Teratol., 4: 177-184.

WALTON, J.N. (1974) Disorders of voluntary muscle, 3rd ed., Edinburg, London, Churchill Livingston.

WANG, G.H. (1932) Relation between spontaneous activity and oestrous cycle in the white rat. Comp. Psychol. Monogr., 6: 1-32.

WEIBEL, E.R. (1979) Stereological methods. In: Practical methods for biological morphometry, New York, Academic Press, Vol. 1.

WEISS, B., FERRIN, J., MERIGAN, M., & COX, C. (1981) Modification of rat operant behaviour by ozone exposure. Toxicol. appl. Pharmacol., 58: 244-251.

WEISS, B. & LATIES, V. (1961) Changes in pain tolerance and other behavior produced by salicylates. J. Pharmacol. exp. Ther., 131: 120-129.

WEISS, B. & LATIES, V. (1969) Behavioral pharmacology and toxicology. Ann. Rev. Pharmacol., 9: 297-326.

WEISS, B. & LATIES, V.G., ed. (1975) Behavioral toxicology, New York, Plenum Press, 469 pp.

WEISS, B. & LATIES, V.G. (1979) Assays for behavioural toxicity: a strategy for the Environmental Protection Agency. Neurobehav. Toxicol., 1(Suppl. 1): 213-215.

WELCH, R.M., LEVIN, W., KUNTZMAN, R., JACOBSON, J., CONNEY, A.H. (1971) Effect of halogenated hydrocarbon insecticides on the metabolism and uterotropic action of estrogens in rats and mice. Toxicol. appl. Pharmacol., 19: 234-246.

WELLS, G.A.H., HOWELL, J.M., & GOPINATH, C. (1976) Experimental lead encephalopathy of calves: histological observations on the nature and distribution of the lesions. Neuropathol. appl. Neurobiol., 2: 175-190.

WHEATLEY, B., BARBEAU, A., CLARKSON, T.W., & LAPHAM, L.W. (1979) Methylmercury poisoning in Canadian indians - the elusive diagnosis. Can. J. neurol. Sci., 6: 417-422.

WHO (1975) Methods used in the USSR for establishing biologically safe levels of toxic substances, Geneva, World Health Organization, 171 pp.

WHO (1978) Principles and methods of evaluating the toxicity of chemicals. Part 1, Geneva, World Health Organization (Environmental Health Criteria Series No. 6, Part 1).

WHO (1984) Principles for evaluating health risks to progeny associated with exposure to chemicals during pregnancy, Geneva, World Health Organization (Environmental Health Criteria Series No. 30).

WHO (in preparation) Principles and methods of evaluating the toxicity of chemicals. Part 2, Geneva, World Health Organization (Environmental Health Criteria Series No. 6, Part 2).

WILLIAMS, P.L. & WARWICK, R. (1975) Functional neuroanatomy of man, Philadelphia, Pennsylvania, W.B. Saunders Company.

WILSON, W.E. (1982) Dopamine-sensitive adenylate cyclase inactivation by organolead compounds. Neurotoxicology, 3: 100-107.

WINNEKE, G. (1979) Modification of visual evoked potentials in rats after long-term blood lead elevation. Act. Nerv. super. (Praha), 21: 282-284.

WINNEKE, G., BROCKHAUS, A., & BALTISSEN, R. (1977) Neurobehavioral and systematic effects of longterm blood lead-elevation in rats. I. Discrimination learning and open field behavior. Arch. Toxicol., 37: 247-263.

WINNEKE, G., FODOR, G., & SCHLIPKOTER, H. (1978) Carbon monoxide, trichloroethylene, and alcohol: reliability and validity of neurobehavioural effects. Multidisciplinary perspectives in event-related brain potentials. In: Proceedings of the Fourth International Congress on Event-Related Slow Potentials of the Brain, Henderson, North Carolina, 4-10 April, 1976 (EPIC IV), Washington DC, US Environmental Protection Agency (EPA 600/9-77-0443).

WINNEKE, G., LILIENTHAL, H., & ZIMMERMANN, U. (1984) Neurobehavioural effects of lead and cadmium. In: Proceedings of the Third International Congress on Toxicology, San Diego, 28 August-2 September 1983, Amsterdam, Oxford, New York, Elsevier Science Publishers.

WOLF, D.L. (1976) Rotating rod, spontaneous activity, and passive avoidance conditioning: their suitability as functional tests in industrial toxicology. In: Horvath, M. & Frantik, E., ed. Adverse effects of environmental chemicals and psycho- tropic drugs, Amsterdam, Oxford, New York, Elsevier Science Publishers, pp. 293-303.

WOOD, R.W. (1978) Stimulus properties of inhaled substances. Environ. Health Perspect., 26: 69-76.

WOOD, R.W. (1979) Reinforcing properties of inhaled substances. Neurobehav. Toxicol., 1(Suppl. 1): 67-72.

WOOD, R.W. (1981) Neurobehavioral toxicity of carbon disulfide. Neurobehav. Toxicol. Teratol., 3: 397-405.

WOOLLEY, D.E. (1977) Electrophysiological techniques in neurotoxicology. In: Zenick, H. & Reiter, L.W., ed. Behavioral toxicology: an emerging discipline, Research Triangle Park, North Carolina, US Environmental Protection Agency, pp. 9-1 - 9-25 (EPA 600/9-77-042).

XINTARAS, C. & BURG, J.R. (1981) Neurotoxicity studies of workers exposed to carbon disulfide. G. Ital. Med. Lav., 3: 83-86.

XINTARAS, C., JOHNSON, B.L., & DEGROOT, I., ed. (1974) Behavioral toxicology, Cincinnati, Ohio, US Department of Health, Education and Welfare, 507 pp (US DHEW (NIOSH) Publication No. 74-126).

YAMAMURA, H.I., ENNA, S.J., & KUHAR, M.J. (1981) Neurotransmitter receptor binding, New York, Raven Press.

YONESAWA, T., BORNSTEIN, M.B., & PETERSON, E.R. (1980) Organotypic cultures of nerve tissue as a model for neurotoxicity investigation and screening. In: Spencer, P.S. & Schaumburg, H.H., ed. Experimental and clinical neurotoxicology, Baltimore, Maryland, Williams and Wilkins Company, pp. 788-802.

YOUNG, J.S. & FECHTER, L.D. (1983) Reflex inhibition procedures for animal audiometry: a technique for assessing ototoxicity. J. Acoust. Soc. Am., 73: 1686-1693.

ZAKUSOV, V.V. (1936) [Estimation of the reflex time under the influence of some narcotic substances.] Fiziol. Zh. USSR, 23: 276-278 (in Russian).

ZAKUSOV, V.V. (1953) [Pharmacology of the nervous system,] Leningrad, Medgiz, 258 pp (in Russian).

ZBINDEN, G. (1981) Experimental methods in behavioral teratology. Arch. Toxicol., 48: 69-88.

ZEMAN, W. & INNES, J.R.M. (1963) Craigie's neuroanatomy of the rat, New York, Academic Press.

ZENICK, H., RODRIQUEZ, W., WARD, J., & ELKINGTON, B. (1979) Deficits in fixed-interval performance following prenatal and postnatal lead exposure. Dev. Psychobiol., 12(5): 509-514.

ZILOV, V.G., ROGACHEVA, S.K., & IVANOVA, L.I. (1983) [Electroencephalographic analysis of limbic-reticular interrelations in various motivational reactions of rabbits under ethanol.] Bull. exp. Biol. Med., 11: 74-77 (in Russian).

ZUBER, V.L. (1978) Intensity of metabolism of various fractions of cerebral phospholipids under hyperphenyl-alaninaemia. Vop. med. Xhim., 2: 163-166.

ZYLBER-HARAN, E.A., GERSHMAN, H., ROSENMANN, E., & SPITZ, I.M. (1982) Gonadotrophin, testosterone, and prolactin interrelationships in cadmium-treated rats. J. Endocrinol., 92: 123-130.

www.ingramcontent.com/pod-product-compliance
Ingram Content Group UK Ltd.
Pitfield, Milton Keynes, MK11 3LW, UK
UKHW021311180426
11947UKWH00015B/1168